ADVANCES IN OSTEOPOROSIS

Edited by **Yannis Dionyssiotis**

Advances in Osteoporosis
http://dx.doi.org/10.5772/58645
Edited by Yannis Dionyssiotis

Contributors

Vinita Mishra, Fahad Alshahrani, Mussa Almalki, Lacramioara Ochiuz, Anca Giorgiana Grigoras, Cristina Mihaela Ghiciuc, Tulay Okman-Kilic, Yan Zhang, Jorge Malouf Sierra, Berta Magallares-López, Robert Güerri-Fernández, You-Qiang Song, Mukhtiar Baig, Saba Tariq, Sundus Tariq

Published by InTech

Janeza Trdine 9, 51000 Rijeka, Croatia

Publishing Process Manager Iva Lipovic

Technical Editor InTech DTP team

Cover InTech Design team

First published March, 2015

Printed in Croatia

Additional hard copies can be obtained from orders@intechopen.com

Advances in Osteoporosis, Edited by Yannis Dionyssiotis

p. cm.

ISBN 978-953-51-2027-8

For EU product safety concerns:
IN TECH d.o.o., Prolaz Marije Krucifikse Kozulić 3, 51000 Rijeka, Croatia,
info@intechopen.com or visit our website at intechopen.com.

Meet the editor

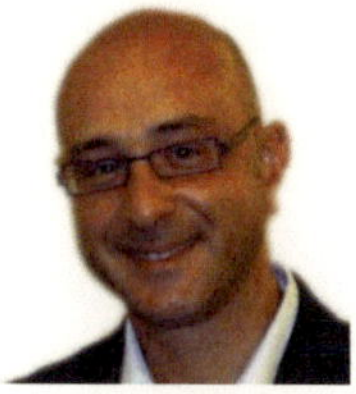

Dr. Yannis Dionyssiotis is specialized in Physical Medicine and Rehabilitation. He has worked as Research Fellow in the Laboratory for Research of the Musculoskeletal System at the University of Athens, as Consultant Physiatrist in the Rehabilitation Department of KAT Hospital in Athens, Head of Physical Medicine and Rehabilitation Department in Rhodes General Hospital and Medical Director of Rehabilitation Center Amyntaio of Florina General Hospital in Greece, and as Stationsarzt in the Klinik für neuro-chirourgische/logische Frührehabilitation, Westpfalz-Klinikum in Germany. Currently, he is the Medical Director of Physical Medicine and Rehabilitation Department of European Interbalkan Medical Center in Thessaloniki and is also working as Research Fellow in the 1st Department of Orthopaedics in General University Hospital ATTIKON. Dr. Dionyssiotis has clinical experience as physiatrist including experience in a variety of clinical settings as clinician, researcher, clinical instructor and consultant. He also holds a Thesis in Osteoporosis and Metabolic Bone Diseases from National and Kapodistrian University of Athens. Dr. Dionyssiotis has an extensive list of professional presentations and publications in the areas of rehabilitation, spinal cord injury, multiple sclerosis and osteoporosis. He has served as reviewer for several international, pubmed and peer-reviewed journals.

Contents

Preface

A balanced regulation of bone formation and resorption in the healthy individual is required for a healthy bone. On the other side, there are many factors which can lead to alterations in bone density and microarchitecture. Menopause is a condition which can increase the remodeling process in favor of resorption. Moreover, there are also some diseases, i.e. chronic kidney bone disease, that increase the possibility of fractures and the subsequent disability leading to increased mortality. However, it is clear that drugs are an essential element of the therapy and this issue is analyzed extensively in this book. Some novel pathophysiological mechanisms are also presented, offering advanced knowledge to the reader.

The book includes chapters from scientific departments and researchers from all over the world. It was my pleasure to edit this book written by experts in the field. Finally, I would like to thank InTech for its contribution to world's scientific knowledge.

Yannis Dionyssiotis, MD, PhD
Physical Medicine and Rehabilitation Physician
Med. Dir. European Interbalkan Medical Center,
Thessaloniki,
Greece

Chapter 1

Densitometric Diagnosis Of Osteoporosis

Fahad M. Alshahrani and Mussa H. Almalki

Additional information is available at the end of the chapter

http://dx.doi.org/10.5772/59437

1. Introduction

Previously, osteoporosis was diagnosed as an absolute decrease in the amount of bone and fracture after minimal trauma[1]. The disadvantage with this definition is patients already have fractures and osteoporosis is sufficiently advanced for it to be visualized on the plain X-ray. The National Institute of Health (NIH) has redefined osteoporosis as a skeletal disorder characterized by compromised bone strength that increases the risk of fracture[2]. Bone strength primarily reflects the integration of bone density and bone quality. Bone quality refers to architecture, turnover, damage accumulation and mineralization. Currently there is no accurate measure of the overall bone quality. The ability to precisely measure bone mineral density (BMD) has only become available in the past few decades and accounts for approximately 70% of bone strength [3,4].

2. Bone densitometry

Traditional X-rays cannot measure bone density, however, they may provide suggestive evidence of osteoporosis. However, this is not accurate and BMD must be decreased by approximately 50% to be appreciated on a plain X-ray. Moreover, radiologist subjective assessments are not always correct. Therefore, routine X-rays are not intended to assess BMD and an apparently normal appearance cannot exclude osteoporosis.[5] Dual-energy X-ray absorptiometry (DXA, previously DEXA[6, 7]), designed to determine bone minerals in central sites such as lumbar spine and the hip, is of greater relevance to clinical osteoporosis. Sometimes forearm measurements can also be made, but they are not routine. Central DXA examinations have three major roles, namely the diagnosis of osteoporosis, the assessment of patients' risk of fracture, and monitoring the response to treatment. Different centres use different machines with different software that make it imperative to perform the follow up on the same machine. Usually, DXA gives a precise and accurate measurement of BMD, but under certain conditions this may lead to an over or under estimation[8] (Table1).

Non- osteoporotic causes of low BMD	Falsely high BMD
Osteomalacia	Degenerative change/ arthritis
Osteogenesis imperficta	Vertebral fracture
Renal bone disease	Artefacts
Multiple myeloma	Vertebroplasty
Mastocytosis	Kyphoplasty

Table 1. Pitfalls in Measurements of Bone Mineral Density.

3. Diagnosis of osteoporosis

The DXA report provides the bone mineral content in a given area of bone. This gives a BMD in grams per square centimetre (g/cm^2). However, The BMD values in (g/cm^2) are not used for diagnosing osteoporosis. Instead, a working group of the World Health Organization (WHO) proposed defining osteoporosis on the basis of the T-score measured by the central DXA at the lumbar spine, total hip or femoral neck (or 1/3 radius if the lumber spine or hip cannot be measured) in a postmenopausal woman and men 50 years and older. A BMD T-score that is 2.5 standard deviation or more below the young-adult mean BMD is defined as osteoporosis, provided that the other causes of low BMD have been excluded (such as osteomalacia). (Table2)

Category	*Bone mass*
Normal	A value for BMD within 1 SD of the young adult female reference mean (T-score at -1.0 and above)
Low bone mass "Osteopenia"	A value for BMD of more than 1 but less than 2.5 SD below the young adult female reference mean (T-score between -1.0 and -2.5)
Osteoporosis	A value for BMD of 2.5 or more SD below the young adult female reference mean (T-score at or below -2.5)
Severe (established) osteoporosis	A value for BMD of 2.5 or more SD below the young adult female reference mean in the presence of one or more fragility fractures

Table 2. Diagnostic categories for osteoporosis and low bone mass based upon bone mineral density measurements by DXA.

The WHO group also described a second diagnostic category, which was termed "osteopenia" defined as a T-score between-1.0 and-2.5 standard deviation. Experts are moving away from the term osteopenia and instead simply labelling it as low bone density. However, there are more fractures in this range because there are so many more patients in this category.

A T-score calculated using the formula: (patient's BMD – young normal mean)/SD of young normal (same gender and ethnicity). For example, if a patient has a BMD of 0.700 (g/cm^2), the young normal mean is 1.000(g/cm^2), and the young normal SD is 0.100 (g/cm^2), then this patient's T-score would be (0.700–1.000)/0.100, or −0.300/0.100, or −3.0. A T-score of 0 is equal to the young normal mean value, −1.0 is 1 SD low, and −3.0 is 3 SD low[8]. Usually, 1 SD is equal to 10 to 15 percent of the BMD value in (g/cm^2). In addition to the T-scores, DXA reports also provide Z-scores, which are calculated similarly to the T-score, except that the patient's BMD is compared with an age-matched (race and gender-matched) mean, and the result is expressed as an SD score. Since bone density declines with age, using the Z score for a diagnosis would suggest that the prevalence of osteoporosis does not increase with age.

The WHO classification should not applied to healthy premenopausal women, men less than 50 years of age and children. In these groups, Osteoporosis cannot be diagnosed on the basis of densitometric criteria alone. The international society for clinical densitometry (ISCD) recommends using the Z-scores rather than T-scores. A Z-score of-2.0 or lower is defined as "below the expected range for age" and a Z-score above-2.0 is "within the expected range for age" [9].

Although not part of the WHO classification, a clinical osteoporosis, regardless of T-score, should be considered in the presence of a fragility fracture (that occurs as a result of a minimal trauma, such as a fall from a standing height or less, or no identifiable trauma) particularly at the spine, proximal femur (hip), distal forearm (wrist) and proximal hummers. Provided other causes for fractures have been excluded, such as a motor vehicle accident, pathological fractures and stress fractures. Certain skeletal locations, including the skull, cervical spine, feet and hands are not associated with fragility fractures [7,10].

4. Site of measurement of BMD

The international society for clinical densitometry (ISCD) recommends obtaining BMD measurements of the posteroanterior spine and hip (right or left) in very obese patients, those with primary hyperparathyroidism, or those in whom the hip or the spine, or both, cannot be measured or interpreted such as with degenerative arthritis, prior vertebral fractures, vertebroplasty and total hip arthroplasty, BMD may be measured in the forearm, using a 33% radius on the nondominant forearm by DXA or peripheral DXA[9], otherwise non-central DXA bone mass measurement devices cannot be used for the diagnosis using the WHO classification. However, it may be used to assess fracture risk.

5. Conclusion

Osteoporosis can be diagnosed clinically or radiographically by DXA. BMD assessment by a central DXA scan of the total hip, femoral neck, or lumbar spine is the standard test to diagnose osteoporosis in a postmenopausal woman or men over age 50, based on the WHO classification. A BMD T-score of 2.5 or more below the young-adult mean BMD is defined as osteoporosis. It is appropriate to consider a clinical diagnosis of osteoporosis in individuals who have sustained fragility fracture(s) even if BMD is not in the osteoporotic range, as the majority of fractures occur in those who have a T-score above-2.5. The WHO classification should not be applied to premenopausal women and men less than 50 years of age and children. Z–scores, not T-scores are preferred. A Z-score of-2.0 or lower is defined as "below the expected range for age". However, in these groups osteoporosis cannot be diagnosed on densitometric criteria alone[9].

Author details

Fahad M. Alshahrani[1,3*] and Mussa H. Almalki[2,3]

*Address all correspondence to: fahad_alshahrani@yahoo.com

1 Family Medicine Department, King Abdulaziz Medical City, National Guard, Riyadh, Saudi Arabia

2 King Fahad Medical City, Riyadh, Saudi Arabia

3 Faculty of Medicine, King Saud bin Abdulaziz University for Health Sciences, Saudi Arabia

References

[1] Riggs BL, Melton LJ. Involutional osteoporosis Engl J Med 1986; 314:1676-86.

[2] NIH Consensus Development Panel on Osteoporosis Prevention, Diagnosis, and Therapy. Osteoporosis prevention, diagnosis and therapy. JAMA 2001; 285: 785-795.

[3] Riggs BL, Melton LJ. 3rd. The prevention and treatment of osteoporosis. N Engl J Med 1992; 327:620-7.

[4] Kanis JA, Delmas P, Burckhardt P, Cooper C, Torgerson D. Guidelines for diagnosis and management of osteoporosis. The European Foundation for Osteoporosis and Bone Disease. Osteoporos Int 1997; 7:390-406.

[5] Garton MJ, Robertson EM, Gilbert FJ et al. Can radiologists detect osteoporosis on plain radiographs? Clin Radiol 1994;49:118-22.

[6] Kanis JA, Melton LJ, Christiansen C, Johnston CC, Khaltaev N. The diagnosis of osteoporosis. J Bone Miner Res. 1994; 9(8):1137-1141.

[7] Kanis JA, McCloskey EV, Johansson H, et al. A reference standard for the description of osteoporosis. Bone 2008; 42(3):467-475.

[8] Watts NB. Fundamentals and pitfalls of bone densitometry using dual-energy X-ray absorptiometry (DXA). Osteoporos Int 2004; 15:847-54.

[9] Leslie WD, Adler RA, El-Hajj FG, et al. Application of the 1994 WHO Classification to Populations Other Than Postmenopausal Caucasian Women: The 2005 ISCD Official Positions. J Clin Densitom 2006; 9(1):22-30.

[10] Mauck KF, Clarke BL. Diagnosis, screening, prevention, and treatment of osteoporosis. Mayo Clin Proc. 2006; 81(5):662–672.

Chapter 2

Estrogen Deficiency and Osteoporosis

Tulay Okman-Kilic

Additional information is available at the end of the chapter

http://dx.doi.org/10.5772/59407

1. Introduction

Estrogen plays a principal role in skeletal growth and bone homeostasis. In women, estrogen deficiency after menopause accelerates frequently osteoclastic bone resorption. It was believed that the accelerated phase in women is most apparent during the first 3 to 5 years after menopause, involved unproportional loss of trabecular bone [1].

We know that the mechanisms of how estrogen deficiency causes bone losses are complex. Researches during the last decade have demonstrated that estrogen regulates bone homeostasis through unexpected regulatory effects on the immune system and on oxidative stres and direct effects on bone cells [2].

We review how the differential effects of estrogen on cortical and trabecular bone might occur and how estrogen might interact with other age-related processes. Estrogen has three fundamental effects on bone metabolism:

1. It inhibits the activation of bone remodeling and the initiation of new basic multicellular units (BMUs);

2. It inhibits differentiation and promotes apoptosis of osteoclasts, therefore bone resorption reduces and

3. While estrogen suppresses self-regeneration of early mesenchymal progenitors, it organizes the commitment and differentiation and prevents apoptosis of osteoblastic cells, therefore bone formation is maintaining at the cellular level [1].

In this review, we summarized each of these actions of estrogen Figure 1,2.

2. The effects of estrogen on the bone cells

At the tissue level, estrogen reduces bone turnover [4]. It would appear that osteocytes may regulate the activation of bone remodeling via connections with bone lining cells [5]. It is likely that the antiremodeling effects of estrogen are mediated via the osteocyte. Osteocytes are cells embedded within the bone matrix, derived from the osteoblast that helps to bone remodeling. The bone lining cells comprise a subpopulation of the osteoblast family. These cells are related with the bone surface at sites where a thin no mineralized collagen layer is present. The bone lining cells migrate to form a canopy over the remodeling area, especially at sites adjacent to osteoclasts [6,7]. Indeed, withdrawal of estrogen is associated with increased apoptosis of osteocytes in humans [8]. Recent studies have reported that serum estradiol levels are inversely associated with serum levels of the key inhibitor of Wnt signaling produced by osteocytes, sclerostin, and estrogen treatment of postmenopausal women reduces circulating sclerostin levels [9,10]. Moreover, it has been suggested that Wnt/β-catenin signaling is important to respond to mechanical strain of the osteocyte, and this response also depends on estrogen receptor α (ERα). Wnt signaling is interrupted in the mesenchyme, osteoblast differantiation is reduced and the skeletal development is affected [11]. Thus there is a likely important argument between estrogen and Wnt signaling pathways mediated by the osteocyte [1] Figure 1.

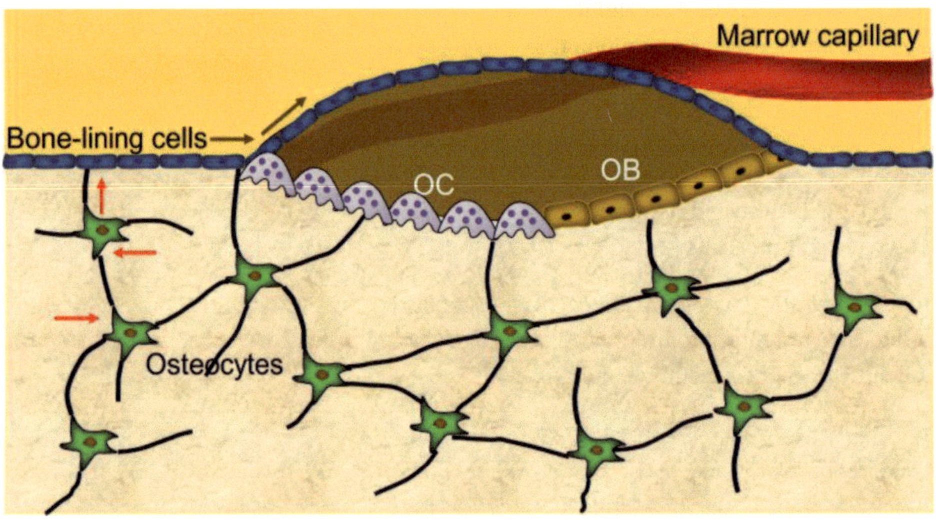

Figure 1. Schematic of the bone remodeling compartment [3] The bone remodeling compartment (BRC) consists of the cells comprising the basic multicellular unit (BMU)-osteoclasts (OCs), osteoblasts (OBs), and osteocytes-as well as the cover bone-lining cells and capillary. These cells are connected with gap junctions. Note also the potential direct physical contact between OCs and OBs, which would allow for signaling between these cells [3].

Estrogen suppresses both directly and indirectly bone resorption [1]. The dominant acute effect of estrogen is blocking the new osteoclast formation. In addition, estrogen also modulates RANK (Receptor activator of nuclear factor κB) signaling in osteoclastic cells [12,13] and induces apoptosis of osteoclasts [14,15]. Osteoclasts are cells of hematopoietic origin responsible for resorbing bone. These are originated from proliferation that occurs by cytokines and differantiation of the monocyte precursors. They are located on endosteal surfaces within the Haversian system and on the periosteal surface [7].

Osteoclast differantiation is supported by cells of the osteoblast lineage. Osteoblast lineage cells consist of osteoblasts, osteocytes and bone lining cells [7]. Osteoclast differantiation process is facilitated by stromal cells of bone marrow that provides physical support to immature OCs. The basic cytokines, need to OC formation under basal conditions are RANKL (Receptor activator of nuclear factor kappa-B ligand) and M-CSF (Macrophage colony-stimulating factor). These factors are produced by major stromal cells of bone marrow, OBs and active T cells. RANKL is a TNF superfamily member. RANKL links transmembrane receptor RANK expressed from OC surface and OC precursors. RANKL also links OPG (Osteoprotegerin), a soluble fake receptor produced by several hemapoietic cells. Therefore OPG functions as an power antiosteoclastogenic cytokine, secreting RANKL and blocking its binding to RANK. RANKL promotes differantiation of OC precursors from early stage of maturation to full maturation (multinucleated OCs) [16] Figure 2.

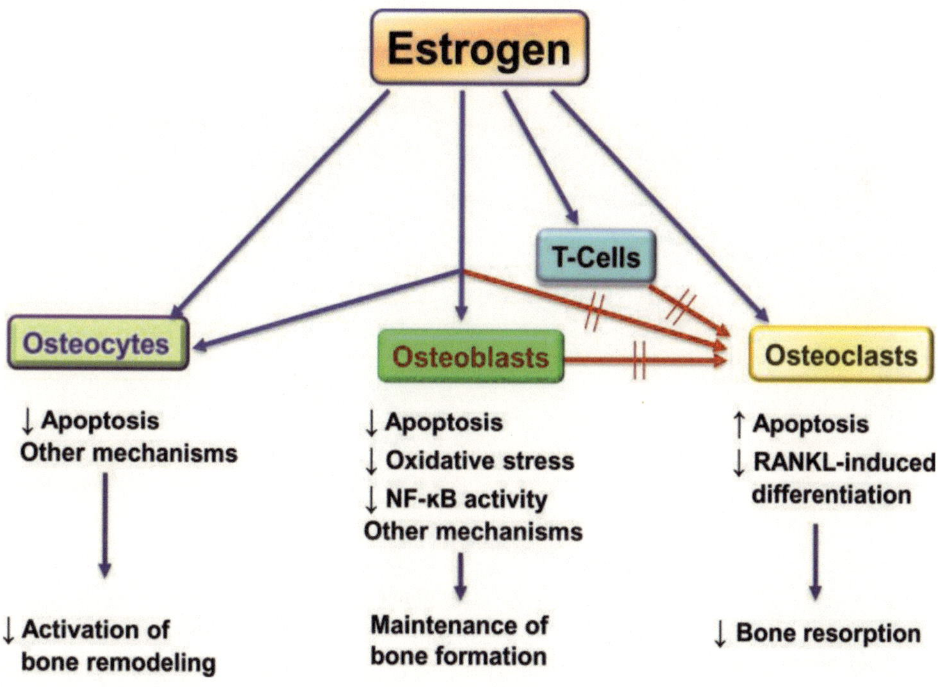

Figure 2. Working model for estrogen regulation of bone turnover via effects on osteocytes, osteoblasts, osteoclasts, and T-cells [3] The main effect of estrogen is inhibition of bone remodeling, likely via the osteocyte. Estrogen also inhibits bone resorption, by direct effects on osteoclasts, although effects of estrogen on osteoblast/osteocyte and T cell regulation of osteoclasts likely also play a role. Estrogen deficiency associated with a gap between bone resorption and formation, likely due to the loss of the effects of estrogen on decreasing osteoblast apoptosis, oxidative stres, osteoblastic NF-κB activity, and perhaps other, as yet undefined mechanisms [3].

Detection of molecular mekanisms that are regulate the osteoclast formation and activation won a big acceleration by survey of RANK/RANKL signal system. M-CSF expression that is secreted by osteoblastic stromal cells need to differentiation to osteoclasts of progenitor cells but, M-CSF expression is not itself sufficient to differentiation of osteoclast. RANKL ekspression by osteoblastic stromal cells and RANK expression by osteoclast precursors need to be completed osteoclast differentiation [17] Figure 3.

Osteoblasts are cell of mesenchymal origin responsible for forming bone. These cells are found along the bone surface at sites of active bone formation. The principal function of the osteoblasts is bone formation [17].

Finally, estrogen is important for the maintenance of bone formation. Human studies show that acute (3 weeks) estrogen deficiency [18] is associated with a fall in bone-formation markers. Chronically estrogen deficient increased both bone-resorption and bone-formation markers [19]. It also appears that the effects of estrogen on progenitor and osteoblastic cells may be stage-specific. Thus, estrogen reduces the self-innovation of early mesenchymal progenitors [20].

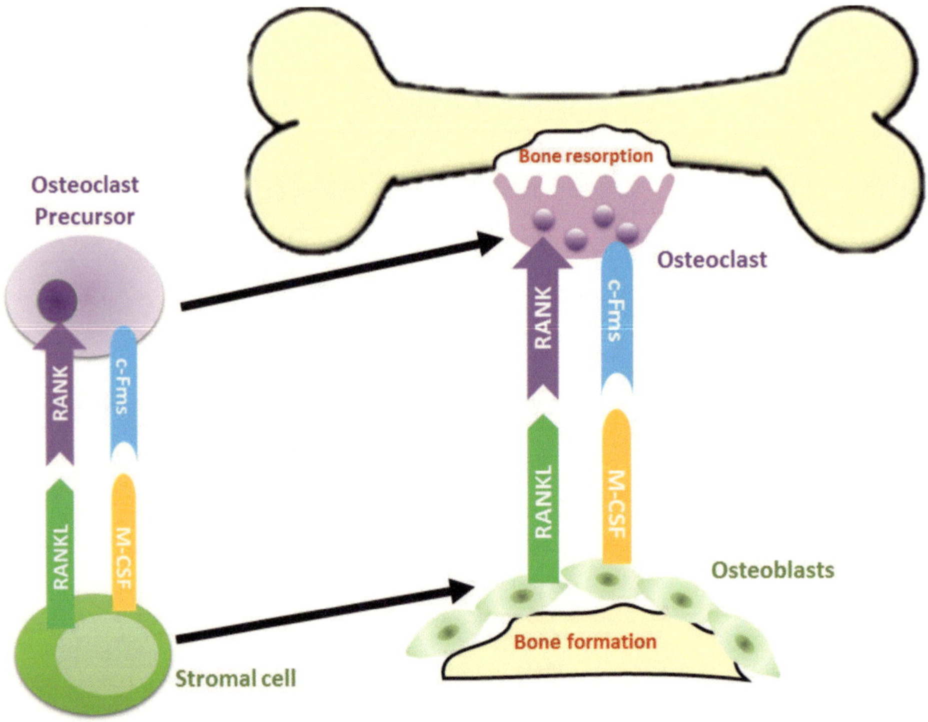

Figure 3. Cells and cytokines responsible for physiological OC renewal. OC precursors may differentiate from the population of monocytes/macrophages. When RANKL binds to receptor RANK in the presence of the trophic factor M-CSF, which in turn binds to its receptor, colony-stimulating factor receptor 1 (c-Fms), OC precursors differentiate and fuse together to multinucleated bone-resorbing OCs. Under physiological conditions the dominant source of RANKL and M-CSF in the bone marrow microenvironment is from the bone-forming cells, the OBs, and their stromal cell (SC) precursors.

It was reported that osteoblasts, osteocytes and osteoclasts express functional estrogen receptors (ERs). These receptors are also expressed in bone marrow stromal cells (SCs), the precursors of osteoblasts [21-24]. Estrogen signals through two receptors, ERalpha and beta [21]. Bone cells contain both receptors, but their distributions within bone are not homogeneous. In hümans, ER alpha is the predominant in cortical bone, but ER beta is predominant in trabecular bone. Although many estrogenic effects are mediated by nuclear ERs, some effects originate in the plazma membrane. Estrogen produces rapid effects in various cell types such as bone cells. These nongenomic effects are due to signaling by a membrane receptor. The induce OC apoptosis and inhibit OB apoptosis of estrogen is linked to its ability to increase ERK1 and ERK2 phosphorylation and repression c-jun N-terminal kinase (JNK) activity [25,26].

It is well recognized that c-jun N-terminal kinases (JNKs) play important roles in cellular functions such as proliferation, differentiation, and cell death in a variety of cell types [24]. JNK activity is essential for the late-stage differentiation of osteoblasts [22].

Extracellular signal-regulated kinase 1 (ERK1) and ERK2 play essential roles in the lineage specification of mesenchymal cells. Inactivation of ERK1 and ERK2 significantly reduced RANKL expression, accounting for a delay in osteoclast formation. ERK1 and ERK2 not only play essential roles in the lineage specification of osteo-chondroprogenitor cells but also support osteoclast formation in vivo [27]. The phosphorylation of these cytoplasmic kinases and their transport to the nucleus modulates the activity transcription factors required for antiapoptotic actions of estrogen [16,26].

3. Estrogen loss and immune system

The immune system plays an important role in the pathophysiology of postmenopausal osteoporosis Figure 4. Estrogen deficiency induces bone loss and increases in production of cytokines, such as IL-1, IL-6, and TNFα. These cytokines are well known regulators of the immune system and T cell function [1,6]. The most important cytokine in the context of estrogen deficiency-induced bone loss has been shown to be TNFα produced by bone marrow T lymphocytes. T lymphocytes are stimulated by a complex mechanism involving several cytokines, such as IL-7, IFN-gamma, and TGF-beta [28].

Estrogen deficiency up-regulates TNF-alpha production by T cells through a complex pathway relative to the thymus and bone marrow. TNF-alpha increases OC formation by up-regulating stromal cell production of RANKL and M-CSF [28,29].

Another cytokine involving OC formation is interleukin-7 (IL-7). It has been reported that IL-7 promotes osteoclastogenesis by up-regulating T cell-derived osteoclastogenic cytokines including RANKL [28,30,31].

INFgamma influences OC formation both via direct and indirect effects [32]. It directly blocks OC formation and provides T cell activation inducing antigen presentation [28,33].

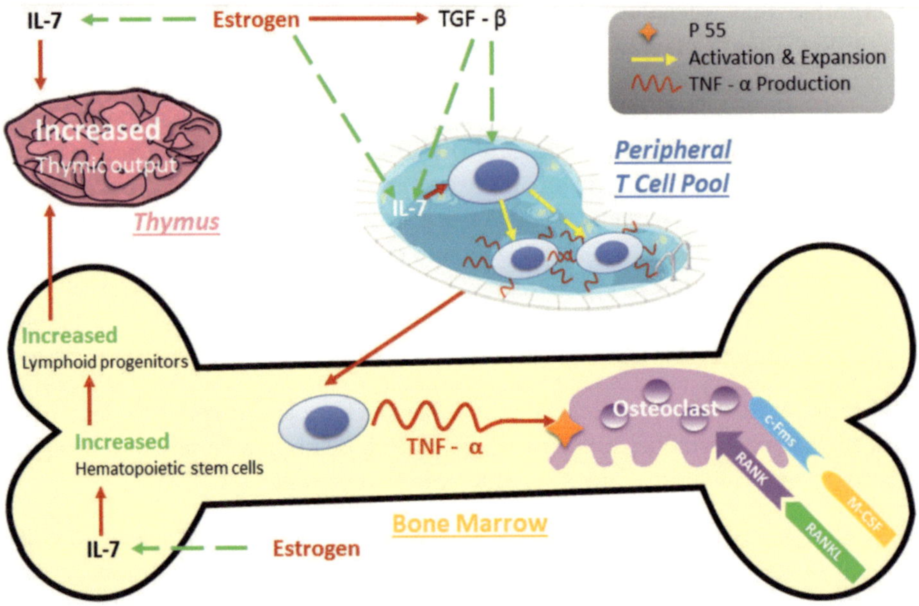

Figure 4. Estrogen suppresses T cell TNF production by regulating T cell differentiation and activity in the bone marrow, thymus, and peripheral lymphoid organs. In the bone marrow, estrogen downregulates the proliferation of hematopoietic stem cells through an IL-7 dependent mechanism. Estrogen prevents T cell activation both directly blunting antigen presentation and via repression of IL-7 and IFN-γ production. This effect is extended by the upregulation of the IL-7 suppressor TGF-β. The net result of them is a decrease in the number of TNF producing T cells. The blunted levels of TNF diminish RANKL-induced OC formation.

Estrogen deficiency induces the imbalance between RANKL and OPG. This situation is important in the occurance of postmenopausal bone loss [34,35].

Recent studies show that postmenopausal wonen have a significantly higher concentration of circulating sclerostin than premenopausal women [28,36]. In vivo and in vitro studies report that TNF-alpha may stimulate the expression of sclerostin. Therefore, the increase of sclerostin mediated by TNF-alpha may contribute to the pathogenesis of postmenopausal women [28,37].

Sclerostin is a protein encoded by the SOST gene in osteocytes. It is a modulator of osteoblast function. Sclerostin antagonizes Wnt signaling and inhibits osteoblastic bone formation [38, 39].

Tyagi et al suggest that Th17 cells may be refer to the pathogenesis of bone loss. Th17 cells produce IL-17. Therefore, IL-17 plays a critical role in Ovx-induced bone loss and may be considered as a potential therapeutic target in pathogenesis of postmenopausal osteoporosis [40].

The thymus undergoes progressive structural and functional decline with age [41]. By middle age most parenchymal tissue is replaced by fat, and fewer T cells are produced, but the thymus progresses to generate new T cells even into old age [16,42,43]. The mechanism of thymic rebound is not completely understood, but may be involving IL-7 [44]. IL-7 alone is not sufficient to enhance thymopoiesis in young mice [45].

Estrogen have suppressive effect on thymic function. Estrogen deficiency induces a rebound in thymic function. Stimulated thymic T cell output accounts for approximately 50% of the increase in the number of T cells in the periphery. Thymectomy also reduces by approximately 50% the bone loss induced by ovariectomy (ovx). This finding shows that estrogen deficiency induced thymic rebound may be responsible for exaggerated bone loss after surgical menopause or in the first 5-7 years after natural menopause [16].

4. Estrogen loss and oxidative stress

In fact, estrogen deficiency accelerates the effects of aging on bone by decreasing defense against oxidative stres (OS). Estrogen protects the adult skeleton against bone loss by slowing the rate of bone remodeling and by maintaining a focal balance between bone formation and resorption. The acut loss of sex steroids shows an increase in the rate of bone remodeling, resulting from an increase in both osteoclastogenesis and osteoblastogenesis [16].

Recent studies report that Reactive oxygen species (ROS) may play a role in postmenopausal bone loss by creating a more oxidized bone microenvironment [46,47] and increase the intracellular concentration of the antioxidant glutathione in bone prevents bone loss during estrogen deficiency in mice [48]. Glutathione peroxidase is responsible for intracellular degradation of hydrogen peroxide. It is the predominant antioxidant enzyme expressed by OCs. Its overexpression abolishes OC formation [49].

Though the mechanisms of ROS action on bone during estrogen deficiency are not well-known, it is reported that immune cells are biological targets of ROS. ROS are important stimulators of antigen presentation by dendritic cell (DC) as well as DC-induced T cell activation [50,51]. ROS are also raised upon dendritic cell interaction with T cells [52]. ROS can decrease T cell lifespan by stimulating T cell apoptosis [53].

It has been shown that NO donor nitroglycerin significantly prevents osteoporotic fractures in postmenopausal women [54] and N-acetyl-cysteine (NAC) treatment prevents against ovx-induced bone loss [48]. NAC treatment blunts ovx-induced dendritic cell activation in the bone marrow, and prevents T cell activation and TNF-alpha production [16].

5. Conclusion

Bone tissue is continually being renewed by osteoclast and osteoblast cells during normal physiology, but excessive resorption occurs without adequate new bone formation during postmenopausal osteoporosis. It has been suggested that such cellular changes are a result of postmenopausal estrogen deficiency. Recent studies report that estrogen deficiency exacerbates bone loss due to aging by diminishing the cells resistance to oxidative stres (OS). Moreover, a relationship between the immune system and bone has been speculated.

Remarkable progression has been registered for our understanding to the mechanisms of bone destruction during estrogen deficiency in the last 2 decades, but additional animal models and long-term human studies are needed.

Future studies will be guide to a new therapeutic advance in the treatment of osteoporosis with a novel mechanism of action that leads to the decrease of bone resorption and fractur risk.

Acknowledgements

The author thanks to Ajlan Okman, for assistance to design of figures.

Author details

Tulay Okman-Kilic*

Address all correspondence to: ajlankilic@hotmail.com

Department of Obsterics and Gynecology, Trakya University, Medical Faculty, Edirne, Turkey

References

[1] Khosla S, Melton LJ 3rd, Riggs BL The unitary model for estrogen deficiency nd the pathogenesis of osteoporosis: is a revision needed? J Bone Miner Res. 2011;26(3): 441-51.

[2] Weitzmann MN, Pacifici R. Estrogen deficiency and bone loss: an inflammatory tale. L Clin Invest. 2006;116(5):1186-94.

[3] Khosla S, Oursler MJ, Monroe DG. Estrogen and the skeleton. Trends Endocrinol Metab. 2012;23(11):576-81.

[4] Lufkin EG, Wahner HW, O'Fallon WM, et al. Treatment of postmenopausal osteoporosis with transdermal estrogen. Ann Intern Med. 1992;117:1–9.

[5] Bonewald LF. Osteocyte messages from a bony tomb. Cell Metab. 2007;5:410–11.

[6] Everts V, Delaisse JM, Korper W, Jansen DC, Tigchelaar-Gutter W, Safting P, et al. The bone lining cell: Its role in cleaning howship's lacunae and initiating bone formation. J Bone Miner Res. 2002;17(1):77-90.

[7] Torres AYP, Flores MV, Orozco L, Cruz RV. Molecular aspects of bone remodeling. In: Flores MV. (ed). Topics in osteoporosis, Rijeka:In Tech; 2013. p1-27.

[8] Tomkinson A, Reeve J, Shaw RW, Noble BS. The death of osteocytes via apoptosis accompanies estrogen withdrawal in human bone. J Clin Endocrinol Metab. 1997;82:3128–35.

[9] Mirza FS, Padhi ID, Raisz LG, Lorenzo JA. Serum sclerostin levels negatively correlate with parathyroid hormone levels and free estrogen index in postmenopausal women. J Clin Endocrinol Metab. 2010;95:1991–97.

[10] Modder UIL, Clowes JA, Hoey K, et al. Regulation of circulating sclerostin levels by sex steroids in women and men. J Bone Miner Res. 2011;26:27–34.

[11] Armstrong VJ, Muzylak M, Sunters A, et al. WNT/B-Catenin signaling is a component of osteoblastic bone cells' early responses to load-bearing, and requires estrogen receptor a. J Biol Chem. 2007;282:20715–27.

[12] Srivastava S, Weitzmann MN, Cenci S, Ross FP, Adler S, Pacifici R. Estrogen decreases TNF gene expression by blocking JNK activity and the resulting production of c-Jun and JunD. J Clin Invest. 1999;104:503–13.

[13] Shevde NK, Bendixen AC, Dienger KM, Pike JW. Estrogens suppress RANK ligand-induced osteoclast differentiation via a stromal cell independent mechanism involving c-Jun repression. Proc Natl Acad Sci USA.2000;97:7829–34.

[14] Nakamura T, Imai Y, Matsumoto T, et al. Estrogen prevents bone loss via estrogen receptor alpha and induction of fas ligand in osteoclasts. Cell. 2007;130:811–23.

[15] Martin-Millan M, Almeida M, Ambrogini E, et al. The estrogen receptor-alpha in osteoclasts mediates the protective effects of estrogens on cancellous but not cortical bone. Mol Endocrinol. 2010;24:323–34.

[16] Weitzmann MN, Pacifici R. Estrogen deficiency and bone loss: an inflammatory tale. J Clin Invest 2006;116(5):1186-94.

[17] Yoshida H, Hayashi S, Kunisada T, Ogawa M, Nishikawa S, Okamura H, Sudo T, Shultz LD. Nature 1990;345:442-44.

[18] Charatcharoenwitthaya N, Khosla S, Atkinson EJ, McCready LK, Riggs BL. Effect of blockade of TNF-a and interleukin-1 action on bone resorption in early postmenopausal women. J Bone Miner Res. 2007;22:724–29.

[19] Garnero P, Sornay-Rendu E, Chapuy M, Delmas PD. Increased bone turnover in late postmenopausal women is a major determinant of osteoporosis. J Bone Miner Res. 1996;11:337–49.

[20] Gregorio GB, Yamamoto M, Ali AA, et al. Attenuation of the self-renewal of transit-amplifying osteoblast progenitors in the murine bone marrow by 17beta-estradiol. J Clin Invest. 2001;107:803–12.

[21] Kuiper G.G, Enmark E, Pelto-Huikko M, Nilsson S and Gustafsson JA. Cloning of a novel receptor expressed in rat prostate and ovary. Proc. Natl. Acad Sci U.S.A. 1996;93:5925-30.

[22] Matsuguchi1T, Chiba N, Bandow K, Kakimoto K, Masuda A, Ohnishi T. JNK activity is essential for Atf4 expression and late-stage osteoblast differentiation. J Bone Miner Res.2009;24:398–410.

[23] Widmann C, Gibson S, Jarpe MB, Johnson GL. Mitogen-activated protein kinase: conservation of a three-kinase module from yeast to human. Physiol Rev. 1999;79: 143–80.

[24] Oursler MJ, Osdoby P, Pyfferoen J, Riggs B, Spelsberg TC. Avian osteoclasts as estrogen target cells. Proc. Natl. Acad. Sci. U. S. A. 1991; 88:6613-17.

[25] Kousteni S, Bellido T, Pilotkin LI, et al. Nongenotropic, sex-nonspecific signaling through the estrogen or androgen receptors: dissociation from transcriptional activity. Cell. 2001;104:719–30.

[26] Kousteni S, Han L, Chen JR, Almeida M, Pilotkin LI, Bellido T, Manolagas SC. Kinase-mediated regulation of common transcription factors accounts for the bone-protective effects of sex steroids. J. Clin. Invest..2003;111:1651–64.

[27] Matsushita T1, Chan YY, Kawanami A, Balmes G, Landreth GE, Murakami S. Extracellular signal-regulated kinase 1 (ERK1) and ERK2 play essential roles in osteoblast differentiation and in supporting osteoclastogenesis. Mol Cell Biol. 2009;(21):5843-57.

[28] Cagnetta V, Patella V. The role of the immune system in the physiopathology pf osteoporosis. Clin cases Miner Bone Metab. 2012;9(2):85-88.

[29] Roato I, Brunetti G, Gorassini E, et al. IL-7 up-regulates TNF-alpha-dependent osteoclastogenesis in patients affected by solid tumor. PLoS One 2006;1:e124.

[30] Toraldo G, Roggia C, Qian WP, et al. IL-7 induces bone loss in vivo by induction of receptor activator of nuclear factor kapa B ligand and tumor necrosis factor alpha from T cells. Proc Natl Acad Sci USA 2003;100:125-30.

[31] Weitzmann MN, Roggia C, Toraldo, et al. Increased production of IL-7 uncoupies bone formation from bone resorption during estrogen deficiency. J Clin Invest 2002;110:1643-50.

[32] Prentice A. Diet, nutrition and the prevention of osteoporosis. Public Health Nutrition. 2004;7:227-43.

[33] Takayanagi H, Kim S, Taniguchi T. Signaling crosstalk between RANKL and interferons in osteoclast differentiation. Artritis Res 2002;4 Suppl 3:227-32.

[34] Hofbauer LC, Khosia S, Dunstan CR, et al. The roles of osteoprotegerin and osteoprotegerin ligand in the paracrine regulation of bone resorption. J Bone Miner Res 2000;15:2-12.

[35] Eghbali-Fatourechi G, Khosia S, Sanyal A, et al. Role of RANK ligand in mediating increased bone resorption in early postmenopausal women. J Clin Invest 2003;111:1221-30.

[36] Mirza FS, Padhi ID, Raisiz LG, and Lorenzo A. Serum sclerostin levels negatively correlate with parathyroid hormone levels and free estrogen index in postmenopausal women. J Clin Endocrinol Metab.2010;95(4):1991-97.

[37] Kim BJ, Bae SJ, Lee SY, Baek JE, Park SY, Lee SH, Koh JM, Kim GS. TNF-alpha mediates the stimulation of sclerostin expression in an estrogen-deficientb condition. Biochem Biophys Res Commun 2012;424(1)170-5.

[38] Okman-Kilic T, Sagiroglu C. Anabolic agents as new treatment strategy in osteoporosis. In: Flores MV. (ed). Topics in osteoporosis, Rijeka: In Tech; 2013. P241-57.

[39] Lewiecki EM. Sclerostin: a novel target for intervention in the treatment of osteoporosis. Discov Med. 2011;12(65):263-73.

[40] Tyagi AM, Srivastava K, Mansoori MN, Trivedi R, Chattopadhyay N, and Singh D. Estrogen deficiency induces the differentiation of IL-17 secreting Th17 cells: a new candidate in the pathogenesis of osteoporosis. PLoS One. 2012;7(9):e44552.

[41] Haynes BF, Sempowski GD, Wells AF, Hale LP. The human thymus during aging. Immunol. Res. 2000;22:253-61.

[42] Douek DC, Koup RA. Evidence for thymic function in the elderly. Vaccine. 2000;18:1638-41.

[43] Jamieson BD, Douek DC, Killian S, Hultin LE, Scripture-Adams DD, Giorgi JV, Marelli D, Koup RA, Zack JA. Generation of functional thymocites in the human adult. Immunity. 1999;10:569-75.

[44] Mackall CL, Fry TJ, Bare C, Morgan P, Galbraith A, Gress RE. IL-7 increases both thymic dependent and thymic independent T cell regeneraion after bone marrow transplantation. Blood. 2001;97:1491-97.

[45] Chu YW, Memon SA, Sharrow SO, Hakim FT, Eckhaus M, Lucas PJ, Gress RE. Exagenous IL-7 increases recent thymic emigrants in peripheral lymphoid tissue without enhanced thymic function. Blood. 2004;104:110-19.

[46] Basu S, Michaelsson K, Olofsson H, Johansson S, Melhus H. Association between oxidative stress and bone mineral density. Biochem. Biophys. Res. Commun 2001;288:275-79.

[47] Maggio D, Barabani M, Pierandrei M, Poliodori MC, Catani M, Mecocci P, Senin U, Pacifici R, Cherubini A. Marked decrease in plasma antioxidants in aged osteoporotic women: results of a cross-sectional study. J Clin Endocrinol Metab. 2003;88:1523-27.

[48] Lean JM, Davies JT, Fuller K, Jagger CJ, Kirstein B, Partington GA, Urry ZL, Chambers TJ. A crucial role for thiol antioxidants in estrogen-deficiency bone loss. J Clin Invest. 2003;112:915-23.

[49] Lean JM, Jagger CJ, Kirstein B, Fuller K, Chambers TJ. Hydrogen peroxide is essential for estrogen deficiency bone loss and osteoclast formation. Endocrinology. 2005;146:728-35.

[50] Mizuashi M, Ohtani T, Nakagawa S, Aiba S. Redox imbalance induced by contact sensitizers tiggers the maturation of dendritic cells. J Invest Dermatol. 2005;124:579-86.

[51] Rutault K, Alderman C, Chain BM, Katz DR. Reactive oxygen species activate human peripheral blood dendritic cells. Free Radic Biol Med. 1999;26:232-38.

[52] Matsue H, Edelbaum D, Shalhevet D, Mizumoto N, Yang C, Mummert ME, Oeda J, Masayasu H, Takashima A. Generation and function of reactive oxygen species in dendritic cells during antigen presentation. J Immunol. 2003;171:3010-18.

[53] Hildeman DA, Mitchell T, Teague TK, Henson P, Day BJ, Kappler J, Marrack PC. Reactive oxygen species regulate activation-induced T cell apoptosis. Immunity. 1999;10:735-44.

[54] Jamal SA, Commings SR, Hawker GA. Isosorbide mononitrate increases bone formation and decreases bone resorption in postmenopausal women: a randomized trial. J Bone Miner Res. 2004;19:1512-17.

Chapter 3

Genetic Disorders Associated with Osteoporosis

Shishu Huang, Gordon Cheung-Toa Ng and
Song You-Qiang

Additional information is available at the end of the chapter

http://dx.doi.org/10.5772/59961

1. Introduction

Osteoporosis (OP) is a common skeletal disease and a global problem. The prevalence of OP is approximately 10.3% in the general population and affects over 200 million women worldwide [1]. Approximately 30% of postmenopausal women suffer from OP in Western nations. About 50% of affected women and at least 15% of affected men will undergo fragility fractures in their lifetime. OP is chronic and does not present with apparent symptoms before osteoporostic fractures occur. This can cause disability, a decreased quality of life, and even death. As a result, OP imposes a heavy financial burden on society that includes not only the direct cost of osteoporostic fractures but also the indirect costs of disablement. In the United States, the direct cost of OP was over USD 13.7 billion in 2005 and may reach USD 25.3 billion by 2025. Therefore, OP is a pressing public health concern and greater understanding of its mechanisms is imperative.

Population ageing is accelerating worldwide, and OP is becoming increasingly prevalent. However, the risk factors that contribute to OP are not clear. Many factors have been suggested to affect the likelihood of OP, including genetics, gender, age, poor diet, smoking and medications (Figure 1). It has been reported that the genetic heritability of bone loss in humans is up to 56% [2,3]. This has been found through comparisons of bone mineral density (BMD), the hallmark trait of OP, in monozygotic (MZ) and dizygotic (DZ) twins after menopause. Additionally, a genome-wide association study (GWAS) of 37,534 individuals in Europe and North America has confirmed that LRP5 (lipoprotein-receptor-related protein) significantly increases the risk of OP and osteoporotic fractures [4]. Therefore, genetic factors play a significant role in the aetiology of OP and its complications.

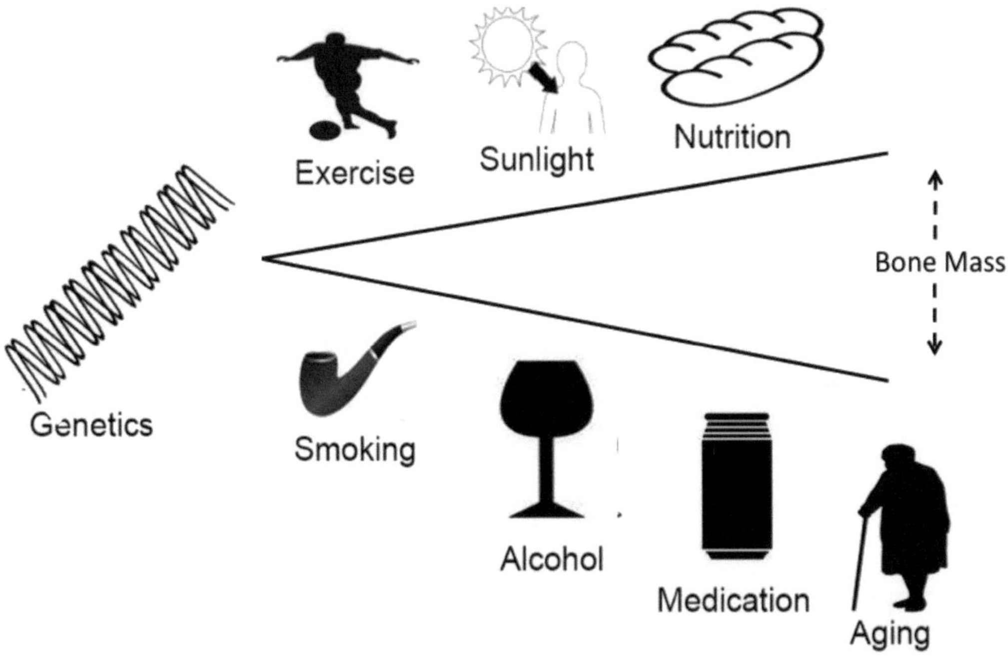

Figure 1. Bone mass is affected by genetic (60%~80% contribution) and other factors (20%~40% contribution) including exercise, sunlight, nutrition, smoking, alcohol, medication and ageing. Factors along the upline potentially contribute to higher bone mass and along the downline cause lower bone mass.

OP is characterized by reduced BMD, impaired microarchitecture of bone tissue and increased risk of fractures. OP has a wide range of phenotypes including abnormal BMD, bone turnover, osteoporotic fracture, skeletal growth, and fracture risk. Although OP genetics aims to identify pathological genes that increase the chance of bone fragility, osteoporotic fractures are not appropriate candidate phenotypes for heritability studies. As fractures occur due to a wide variety of reasons, not necessarily as a result of bone fragility, fractures alone are insufficient qualifiers for studies. In contrast, previous studies have reported a strong genetic correlation between BMD and bone mass/fracture phenotypes [5]. To this date, most OP studies have focused on BMD because of the high heritability and relative ease of measurement. This chapter will discuss the hereditary factors in pursuit of a new understanding of pathological genes in OP, including an overview of current technology at the cutting-edge of OP testing.

2. Non-genetic factors in the risk of osteoporosis

OP may be caused by primary and secondary factors (Table 1). Mostly, OP results from primary factors; in approximately 20%~40% of patients the condition has secondary causes [5,6]. Primary OP has two categories: type I (postmenopausal) and type II (senile) OP. Type I OP is believed to be associated with oestrogen deficiency and usually occurs in women between the ages of 51 and 75. It results in excessive bone resorption and fractures, including in the trabecular bone in the vertebrae and distal radius. Type II OP usually results from age-related vitamin D deficiency and affects women and men over the age of 70. It mainly causes hypocalcaemia, increased parathyroid hormone (PTH) release, bone resorption and fractures, including in both the trabecular and cortical bone on the long bones, causing fractures of the femoral neck, proximal, humerus and tibia, and pelvis.

Identifiable Causes	
Primary cause	***Secondary cause***
Personal condition	Chronic glucocorticoid therapy
Oestrogen deficiency	Thyrotoxicosis
Low weight and body mass index	Vitamin D deficiency
Increased age	Alcoholism and smoking
Gender	Hypogonadism (men)
Family history	Malnutrition

Table 1. Identifiable causes of osteoporosis

As discussed in detail in other chapters of this book, OP is a chronic and complex disease that is influenced by both non-genetic and genetic factors. Non-genetic factors are common and worthy of consideration (Table 2). One of the most important is oestrogen, which changes with age [6, 7]. Oestrogen acts directly on oestrogen receptors in osteoblasts and its deficiency affects BMD, which leads to the risk of OP in postmenopausal women and contributes to the development of OP in elderly men. The chemical element lead is another potential risk factor for OP. Lead impairs cell proliferation and viability by affecting the response of cells to hormonal stimuli, which interferes with hormone and cytokine signal-transduction processes. This causes a toxic effect in skeleton systems and influences bone mineral homeostasis and growth. Calcium is one of our most common body minerals and is required for normal skeletal growth and maintenance [8]. A low-calcium diet causes loss of trabecular bone by affecting the function and phenotype of bone-marrow cells [8-10]. This has been shown to further accelerate bone loss in ovariectomized (OVX) rats, though BMD levels were partially rescued by calcium supplements [8-10]. Cadmium is toxic and causes bone loss after the start of dietary cadmium exposure [11-12]. It has been demonstrated that cadmium exposure leads to an increase in serum calcium, phosphorous and PTH levels in concomitant with significant reduction in serum vitamin D (3), osteocalcin (OC) levels and bone-specific alkaline phosphatase (BALP) activity [11-12]. Reduced BMD is usually associated with kidney impairment in response to cadmium exposure [12]. Although the toxic effects of aluminium overload on bone metabolism were first reported with a severe form of osteomalacic osteodystrophy [13], recently it has been reported that accumulated aluminium content in bone during life does not substantially influence the level of BMD [14-15]. Additionally, no clinical symptoms of bone disease were found in individuals with aluminium contamination, but its accumulation in tissue was significant [14-15]. Interestingly, dual X-ray absorptiometry (DXA) was found to induce BMD recovery in osteopenic rats affected by aluminium [16]. Alcohol slows cell proliferation and viability to arrest longitudinal bone growth, and affects dry weight, mineral content and mechanical integrity [17-18]. This may increase the risk of developing OP – further confirmation is given by epidemiological findings. Additionally, studies on animals have reported that alcohol suppresses young bone growth and inhibits adult bone formation – alcohol has greater deleterious effects on bone formation than on bone resorption [18]. Smoking, particularly heavy smoking, may affect nutritional absorption, decrease absorption of calcium, and interfere with oestrogen. This eventually results in lower oestrogen levels, lower bone density, a dramatic decrease in the bone mass/mineralization, and a higher incidence of bone fractures [19-21]. Notably, smoking duration was not associated with BMD in 1,054 subjects, including 26.2% of current smokers (n=276), 17.7% of former smokers (n=187), and 56.1% of never smokers (n=591) [21].

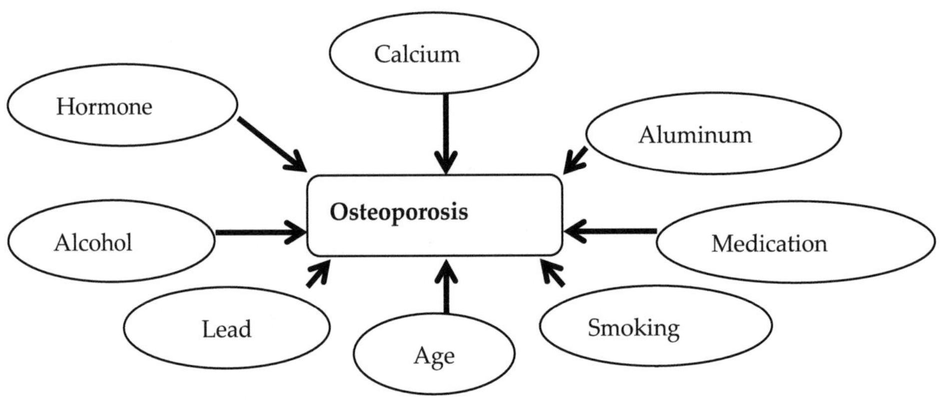

Table 2. Non-genetic factors in the risk of osteoporosis.

Although non-genetic factors play a significant role in determination of the risk of OP, twin and family studies have reported that up to 60~80% of the variance in BMD is attributable to genetic factors. Non-genetic factors vary markedly among individuals who show different bone response to stimuli, and genetic factors appear to be more dominant than the combination of non-genetic factors in the pathogenesis of OP. The search for pathogenic genes that cause OP remains one of the greatest challenges and the most active scientific area in musculoskeletal research. Despite the impact of environmental factors, it has been confirmed that genes related to OP exist and have pathogenicity. These are multiple genes with small individual effects; not more than 10% are associated with BMD. Therefore, the impact of genetic factors in the pathogenesis of OP is still unclear. To date, different methods have been used to identify the susceptible genes related to OP (Fig. 2.). These are elaborated below.

http://dx.doi.org/10.5772/59961

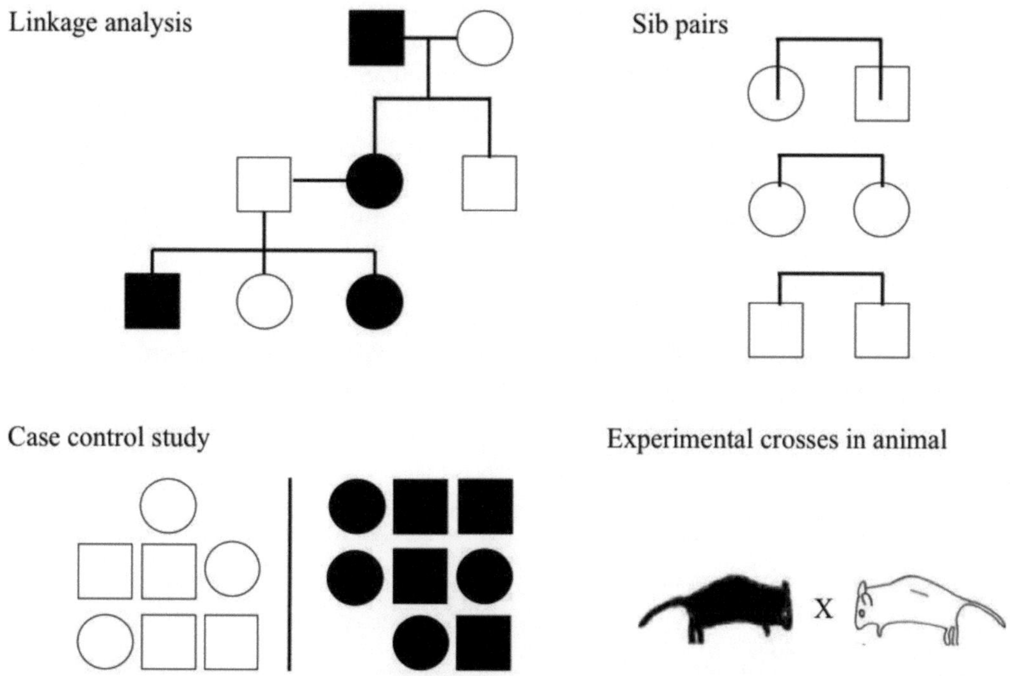

Figure 2. Strategies in the identification of genetic variants of osteoporosis and other complex diseases. Linkage studies in families and sibling pairs refer to phenotyping members of extended families for the feature of interest (e.g., BMD). The control study looks for the association of a marker allele with disease by comparison among unrelated subjects. Experimental crosses in animals are performed to prove the findings from linkage and candidate gene studies.

3. Genes associated with BMD in monogenic skeletal diseases

Ever since Mendel first elucidated the concept of inheritance in the pea plant, genetic analyses have used families, which often share similar genes, to study gene characteristics. With the development of genomic technology, the discovery of genetic markers spanning the entire human genome for Mendelian diseases and traits has been achieved after widespread mapping efforts. Major monogenic skeletal disorders with OP that have been identified to date include osteogenesis imperfecta, Bruck syndrome, osteopetrosis, high-bone-mass syndrome, osteoporosis-pseudoglioma syndrome, von Buchem disease, sclerosteosteosis, familial expansile osteolysis, juvenile Paget's disease, hypophosphatasia, neonatal hyperparathyroidism and pyknodysostosis. These diseases affect BMD and can cause either high- or low-mass syndrome.

Although many pathogenic genes have been identified (Table 3), many do not qualify as osteoporosis genes due to a lack of robustness. Low-density lipoprotein receptor-related 5 (LRP5) protein is a transmembrane low-density lipoprotein receptor which functions in receptor-mediated endocytosis [22-24]. The LRP5 gene was identified as the cause of the monogenic disease osteoporosis-pseudoglioma by mapping and candidate gene screening

[22-24]. Inactivation of LRP5 leads to the suppression of mechano-responsiveness and reduces bone mass and Young's modulus in osteoporosis-pseudoglioma [25, 26]. Activation of LRP5 increases bone mass in osteosarcoma. Furthermore, population-based and cohort studies have confirmed the significant association of LRP5 with BMD in Asian and European populations [27-29]. Bone fragility and risk of fracture have been reported with the mutation of LRP5 in families of affected patients. Patients with multiple thoracic vertebral fractures were confirmed to have about two compound heterozygous missense mutations in LRP5 [30, 31]. Meta-analyses and genome-wide studies carried out for separate large populations have revealed consistency between LRP5 variants in BMD and fracture risk – this will be further addressed in the next part. In addition to LRP5, low-density lipoprotein-related 4 (LRP4) protein was identified as a candidate sclerostin interaction partner by an unbiased proteomics approach [32]. The mutation of LRP4 has been reported to be associated with bone overgrowth by impairing the sclerostin facilitator function.

AR	AHSG	ApoE	BMP2	BGP	CASR
CLCN7	COL1A1	COL1A2	CT	CYR1B1	COMT
CYP1A1	CYP17	CTR	CYP19	CCR2	DBP
DRD4	ERbeta	ERalpha	FRA-1	GH1	GnRH
HLA-A	IL-6	LRP5	LRP4	LCT	IL-1RA
LEPR	IL-10	I-TRAF	IRAK1	IGF-1	IGF-II
Klotho	MMP-1	MGP	MTHFR	MMP-9	NPY
NCOA3	OSCAR	OPG	P57(KIP2)	PON1	PDE4
PPARG	PLDO1	PTHR1	PTH	PDE4D	QPCT
RIL	RUNX2	Sox4	SERT	SOST	TNFalpha
TNFR2	TCIRG1	TGFbeta	WRN		

Table 3. Genes associated with BMD/osteoporosis. These genes are identified through association studies and correlate with BMD and osteoporosis-related phenotype.

Vitamin D receptor (VDR) is one of the trans-acting transcriptional regulatory factors that regulate proteins involved in bone mineral homeostasis. It has been reported that the polymorphism of the third region of VDR is significantly associated with BMD, and the allelic variation of this gene may contribute 75% of the genetic effect on BMD change [33]. Additionally, the polymorphism of the VDR gene, including Bsml, Apal, Fokl and Taq genotypes, regulates BMD and is associated with OP [34-37]. VDR polymorphisms emerge in the rheumatoid-related OP and the ApaI, BsmI and TaqI polymorphisms may be susceptible risk factors for rheumatoid arthritis (RA). Interestingly, the Ff genotype may be responsible for development of OP in RA [38, 39].

Type I collagen is a constituent major-bone protein, and the genes (COLIA1 and COLIA2) are believed to be candidates for genetic control of BMD. The COLIA1 gene polymorphism is suggested to be implicated in reduced BMD and increased fracture incidence [40]. Mutations in the two genes for type I collagen have been confirmed to cause osteogenesis imperfecta, and are associated with OP in postmenopausal women [41, 42]. Population-based studies have indicated that COL1A1 Sp1 polymorphism may contribute to the development of OP such that Sp1 polymorphic variants of COL1A1 gene are associated with BMD values [43-46]. The "ss" and "TT" genotypes possess lower lumbar-spine BMD [46].

The oestrogen-receptor gene encodes an oestrogen receptor (ESR), a member of the super-family of nuclear receptors that are involved in DNA and hormone binding and activation of transcription. The ESR can interact with oestrogen and transcription factors including SP-1, AP-1 and NF-κB. As oestrogens are important endocrine regulators in skeletal growth and maintenance, oestrogen-deficient animals exhibit reduced BMD and oestrogen substitution shows restored bone compartments [47-49]. One case of OP in a male patient was reported to show an inactivating mutation of the ESR gene, which was parallel with the male knockout mice with null alleles at the ESR locus [50]. However, inactivation of ESR alpha, specifically in nervous tissue, the main ER for oestrogenic bone effects, causes increased BMD in mouse trabecular and cortical bone [51]. Interestingly, ER alpha in osteocytes has been shown to play an osteoprotective role in the trabecular bone formation, confirmed by tests on ER alpha-deletion mice [52].

Although many genes have been identified in monogenic skeletal disorders connected to OP, the linkage data have not been sufficiently robust due to sample size and significance. Studies in OP genetics need to facilitate more powerful and more sophisticated approaches, such as GWAS studies, to achieve the identification of OP heritable factors.

4. Genome-wide association study and BMD

Genome-wide association study (GWAS) aims to identify disease-associated loci called single nucleotide polymorphisms (SNPs), which contribute to small variations of BMD in the genome. If an allele of an SNP occurs significantly more or less frequently in people with a particular disease than in people without the disease, the allele is associated with the disease traits. Although previous linkage and candidate-gene studies have provided few replicated loci for OP, genome-wide association approaches have produced clear and reproducible findings.

Two SNPs, rs3736228 on chromosome 11 in the LRP5 gene and rs4355801 on chromosome 8 near the TNFRSF11B gene, were reported to cause risk of OP and osteoporotic fracture in 2,094 British women [53]. The rs3736228 in the LRP5 gene was identified to correlate with decreased BMD in lumbar spine and femoral neck. The rs4355801 near the TNFRSF11B gene correlated with decreased BMD for lumbar spine and femoral neck [53]. In a study of 583 postmenopausal women, the polymorphism of three variants TNFRSF11B (rs4355801, rs2073618, and rs6993813) and one of LRP5 (rs3736228) was further confirmed to be associated with BMD variations [54]. In a prospective study of 37,534 subjects in Europe and North America, variants of LRP5 (rs3736228, rs4988321) and one variant of LRP6 (rs2302685) were examined in terms of their effect on BMD and contribution to risk of fracture. The rs3736228 and rs4988321 variants of LRP5 were associated with reduced lumbar-spine BMD, femoral-neck BMD, and fractures. The rs2302685 of LRP6 polymorphism was not associated with any OP phenotype, including reduced BMD and fracture [55, 56]. This was further confirmed in a study of 944 postmenopausal Spanish women, where the rs2302685 variant of the LRP6 polymorphism was not significantly associated with lumbar-spine or femoral-neck BMD [57]. LRP4 was also analysed for SNP in cohort studies of European populations. One associated SNP of LRP4 (rs6485702) was significant in hip and whole-body BMD, modulated through the Wnt and BMP signalling pathways [58, 59].

Other gene polymorphisms associated with changes in BMD included the Cerberus 1 (CER1) gene, ADAM metallopeptidase with thrombospondin type 1 motif 18 (ADAMTS18), transforming growth factor beta receptor III (TGFBR3), high-mobility group (HMG), signal transducer and activator of transcription 1 (STAT1), aldehyde dehydrogenase (ALDH), PTH, and sperm-ion channel gene CatSper channel auxiliary subunit beta (CATSPERB). In a cohort of 1,083 human subjects, one SNP (rs3747532) in human CER1 gene was reported to play a role in the increased risk of low BMD in women prior to menopause and a vertebral fractures cohort [60]. In an association test of 379,319 SNPs in 1,000 unrelated American white individuals, ADAMTS18 and TGFBR3 were reported as BMD candidate genes in meta-analyses [61]. Additionally, individuals with normal skeletal fractures were different to individuals with non-union skeletal fracture in the expression of both genes [61]. In two cohorts of 1,548 Caucasian American men and 1,680 Afro-Caribbean men, the rs1042725 of the HMGA2 polymorphism was reported to be associated with decreased tibia trabecular volumetric BMD [62]. In a GWAS of 1,000 unrelated Caucasians, the STAT1 gene was significantly associated with BMD variation and was upregulated in the low BMD group rather than the high BMD group variation [63]. In a study of 700 elderly Chinese Han individuals (350 with hip osteoporotic fracture and 350 healthy controls), one SNP, rs13182402, within the ALDH7A1 gene on chromosome 5q31, was significantly associated with osteoporotic fractures [64]. This was further examined in relation to the relevance of hip BMD in Caucasian and Chinese populations (n=9,962), finding a consistent association with hip BMD [64]. The Interleukin 21 receptor (IL21R) encodes a cytokine receptor for interleukin 21 that activates multiple downstream signalling molecules, including STAT1, STAT3, JAK1 and JAK3. In a GWAS of 983 unrelated white subjects, the polymorphisms of the PTH gene (rs9630182, rs2036417, and rs7125774) and the polymorphisms of the IL21R gene (rs7199138, rs8061992 and rs8057551) were associated with changed femoral-neck BMD [65]. The polymorphisms of CATSPERB (rs1298989, rs1285635) were reported to be associated with femoral-neck BMD in 1,524 European-American premenopausal women and 669 African-American premenopausal women [66]. In particular, the rs1285635 in the European-American women was consistent with that in the African-American women [66].

Furthermore, meta-analysis of GWAS has shown more candidate genes and BMD loci reaching genome-wide significance. A meta-analysis of 19,195 Northern European subjects from five GWAS revealed nine genes from 150 identified genes associated with changed BMD: TNFSF11, TNFRSF11A, TNFRSF11B, LRP4, LRP5, ESR1, SPP1, ITGA1, and SOST [67]. Additionally, 13 new BMD loci were identified and included: 1p31.3 (GPR177), 2p21 (SPTBN1), 3p22 (CTNNB1), 4q21.1 (MEPE), 5q14 (MEF2C), 7p14 (STARD3NL), 7q21.3 (FLJ42280), 11p11.2 (LRP4, ARHGAP1, F2), 11p14.1 (DCDC5), 11p15 (SOX6), 16q24 (FOXL1), 17q21 (HDAC5) and 17q12 (CRHR1) [68]. In a meta-analysis of 18,098 subjects from six European-descent populations and an Asian population, rs2273061 of the Jagged1 (JAG1) gene was identified to be associated with BMD for lumbar spine and for femoral neck. The JAG1 gene therefore becomes a new candidate gene in the regulation of BMD and a new risk factor for bone-fracture pathogenesis [69]. In a meta-analysis of GWAS based on 3,657 Caucasian men and 7,633 Caucasian women, two genes and three new loci were identified as associated with OP-related traits and BMD in women, including SOX6, GPR177 gene, 2q11.2 (TBC1D8), chromosome 1p13.2 and 18q11.2 (OSBPL1A) [70]. A meta-analysis of GWAS data from European and Chinese individuals identified further genes associated with changed BMD located at 1q21.3, 9q22, 9q33.2, 20p13, and 20q12. This significantly correlates with the development and functionality of muscle, skeleton and connective tissue [71]. In a meta-analysis of 17 GWAS based on 32,961 subjects of East-Asian and European ancestry, 32 new loci were associated with BMD at genome-wide significance and were localized in 1q24.3, 2p21, 2q13, 2q14.2, 3q13.2, 3q25.31, 4p16.3, 6p21.1, 6p22.3, 7q31.31, 7q31.31, 7q36.1, 8q13.3, 9q34.11, 10p11.23, 10q21.1, 10q22.3_1, 10q24.2, 11p14.1_1, 12p11.22, 12p13.33, 12q13.12, 12q23.3, 14q32.12, 16p13.11, 16p13.3_1, 16p13.3_2, 16q12.1, 17p13.3, 17q24.3, 18p11.21, 19q13.11 and Xp22.31 [72]. Moreover, in a meta-analysis of 27,061 individuals, two new loci were of genome-wide significance: 14q24.2 (rs227425, SMOC1) in the whole sample and 21q22.13 (rs170183, CLDN14) in the female-specific sample. These were also shown to be significant in the results of the GEnetic Factors for Osteoporosis Consortium (GEFOS, n = 32,960) [73].

Thus, GWAS has been successfully used in uncovering key genes or markers associated with OP in humans and animals. Although it has confirmed the existence of relevant SNPs associated with changed BMD and the risk of OP, GWAS still cannot be absolutely accurate in the prediction of OP.

5. Genome-wide copy-number variants study and BMD

The first large-scale genome-wide studies of copy-number variants (CNVs) in humans were performed about a decade ago, and CNVs now make a larger contribution to genome variations than SNPs [74, 75]. Recent studies have focused on CNVs that may modulate gene function and affect disease risk. CNVs are structural genetic variants in the genome that alter the number of copies of one or more sections of DNA. This corresponds to large regions of the genome with deletion or duplication on certain chromosomes, and results in phenotypic variation.

Although CNV has been reported to correlate with many complex human diseases, the contribution of CNV to OP has not been revealed yet. A Chinese study of 700 elderly patients, comprising 350 individuals with homogeneous hip osteoporostic fracture and 350 control individuals, reported that CNV 4q13.2 significantly correlated with osteoporostic fracture

(P<0.0002). Additionally, a variant of UGT2B17 in CNV 4q13.2 was further proven to correlate with hip osteoporostic fracture in both white (1000 individuals) and Chinese (689 individuals), with consistently significant results (P=0.0005-0.021) [76].

Another genome-wide study of 1,000 Caucasian individuals found that a CNV in VPS13B gene, encoding a potential transmembrane protein involved in vesicle-mediated transport, was significantly associated with hip, spine and femoral-neck BMD. Interestingly, individuals with two copies of the CNV in the genome exhibited a higher level of BMD in the hip, spine and femoral neck, compared with one-copy subjects [77].

Another genome-wide CNV study tested 5,178 subjects in a prospective cohort in the Netherlands. It identified 210 kb deletion located on chromosome 6p25.1 that correlated with the risk of fracture (P=0.0000869). This deletion has geographic specificity, not affecting the populations of Australia, Canada, Poland, Iceland, Denmark, or Sweden. It has been found and is prevalent in Ireland (0.06%), England (0.15%), USA (0.23%), Scotland (0.10%), and Spain (0.33%), with insufficient significance of fracture risk. However, the role of the 6p25.1 locus in the prediction of risk of bone fracture needs to be tested in a larger and more diverse population to confirm the findings [78].

A study on 2,286 Caucasian individuals, and replicated in 1,627 Chinese individuals, identified two CNVs (CNV2580 and CNV1191) that correlated with appendicular lean mass (ALM), the main component of skeletal muscle. CNV1191 resides in the gene encoding GTPase of the immunity-associated protein family (GIMAP1), and is significantly associated with ALM (P=0.0226). CNV2580 is localized in the serine hydrolase-like protein (SERHL) gene and is also significantly associated with ALM (P=0.00334). Both genes are important for skeletal-muscle growth and may be relevant to OP. Although the two new CNVs are responsible for variation in ALM, more evidence is required to confirm their significance in relation to OP [79].

Therefore, the use of CNV-based GWAS in relation to OP is a cutting-edge technology and strongly supports the importance of CNV in the pathogenesis of OP. Although the results in this area are well established, it is necessary to focus on the association between classical genotypes, and actual experimentation is needed for validation. Additionally, high-throughput, sophisticated genotyping approaches for CNVs need to be optimized for further genetic screening.

6. Conclusion

OP is one of the most common diseases and is becoming more prevalent with the ageing of the world's population. BMD is the hallmark of OP and exhibits high heritability; efforts to understand OP genetic determinants have therefore been increased. OP represents a paradigm where the effects of multiple genetic factors dominate the phenotype. Although monogenic approaches that identify genes by rare mutations have contributed to the understanding of OP, the genetic background of OP is characterized by polymorphisms and variations in multiple genes; more-powerful and high-throughput technologies are needed to analyse these aspects. Recent genetic studies in OP have facilitated the understanding of the aetiology of OP. The discovery of novel genetic factors through the use of genome sequencing will contribute to understanding the modulation of BMD and bone fragility with potential therapeutic targets. Combined with behavioural and environmental factors, findings in genetic studies can be validated and used in the development of clinical treatments of OP worldwide. There is no doubt that genetic tests have achieved significant progress in bone biology and are likely to become even more important within the next decade. To optimize accuracy, we should highlight elements including careful phenotyping, sophisticated study design, adequately powered cohorts, and multi-collaboration in future research.

Acknowledgements

This study was supported by the Seeding Fund of the Shandong Academy of Sciences, China, Natural Science Foundation of China (81201405, 31470904, 81472078) and the Basic Research Project of Shenzhen (JCYJ20120615125154107).

Author details

Shishu Huang[1,2], Gordon Cheung-Toa Ng[3] and Song You-Qiang[3*]

*Address all correspondence to: songy@hku.hk

1 State Key Laboratory of Oral Diseases, West China College of Stomatology, Sichuan University, PRC

2 Department of Orthopaedics and Traumatology, The University of Hong Kong, PRC

3 Department of Biochemistry, The University of Hong Kong, Pokfulam, Hong Kong SAR, PRC

References

[1] Wright NC, Looker AC, Saag KG, Curtis JR, Delzell ES, Randall S, et al. The Recent Prevalence of Osteoporosis and Low Bone Mass in the United States Based on Bone Mineral Density at the Femoral Neck or Lumbar Spine. Journal of Bone and Mineral Research. 2014. doi: 10.1002/jbmr.2269.

[2] Zhai G, Andrew T, Kato B, Blake G, Spector T. Genetic and environmental determinants on bone loss in postmenopausal Caucasian women: a 14-year longitudinal twin study. Osteoporosis International. 2009;20(6):949-53.

[3] Makovey J, Nguyen TV, Naganathan V, Wark JD, Sambrook PN. Genetic Effects on Bone Loss in Peri- and Postmenopausal Women: A Longitudinal Twin Study. Journal of Bone and Mineral Research. 2007;22(11):1773-80.

[4] Van Meurs JB, Trikalinos TA, Ralston SH, Balcells S, Brandi ML, Brixen K, et al. Large-scale analysis of association between LRP5 and LRP6 variants and osteoporosis. AMA. 2008 Mar 19;299(11):1277-90.

[5] Hernandez-de Sosa N, Athanasiadis G, Malouf J, Laiz A, Marin A, Herrera S, et al. Heritability of Bone Mineral Density in a Multivariate Family-Based Study. Calcified Tissue International. 2014;94(6):590-6.

[6] Richelson LS, Wahner HW, Melton III L, Riggs BL. Relative contributions of aging and estrogen deficiency to postmenopausal bone loss. New England Journal of Medicine. 1984;311(20):1273-5.

[7] Melville KM, Kelly NH, Khan SA, Schimenti JC, Ross FP, Main RP, et al. Female Mice Lacking Estrogen Receptor-Alpha in Osteoblasts Have Compromised Bone Mass and Strength. Journal of Bone and Mineral Research. 2014;29(2):370-9.

[8] Seto H, Aoki K, Kasugai S, Ohya K. Trabecular bone turnover, bone marrow cell development, and gene expression of bone matrix proteins after low calcium feeding in rats. Bone. 1999;25(6):687-95.

[9] Gao X, Ma W, Dong H, Yong Z, Su R. Establishing a rapid animal model of osteoporosis with ovariectomy plus low calcium diet in rats. International Journal of Clinical and Experimental Pathology. 2014;7(8):5123.

[10] Gala J, Piedra CDL, Calero J. Short-and long-term effects of calcium and exercise on bone mineral density in ovariectomized rats. British Journal of Nutrition. 2001;86(04): 521-7.

[11] Youness ER, Mohammed NA, Morsy FA. Cadmium impact and osteoporosis: mechanism of action. Toxicology Mechanisms and Methods. 2012;22(7):560-7.

[12] Chen X, Zhu G, Jin T, Lei L, Liang Y. Bone mineral density is related with previous renal dysfunction caused by cadmium exposure. Environmental Toxicology and Pharmacology. 2011;32(1):46-53.

[13] Ward M, Ellis H, Feest T, Parkinson I, Kerr D, Herrington J, et al. Osteomalacic dialysis osteodystrophy: Evidence for a water-borne aetiological agent, probably aluminium. The Lancet. 1978;311(8069):841-5.

[14] Hellström H-O, Mjöberg B, Mallmin H, Michaëlsson K. No association between the aluminium content of trabecular bone and bone density, mass or size of the proximal femur in elderly men and women. BMC Musculoskeletal Disorders. 2006;7(1):69.

[15] Advenier E, Landry C, Colomb V, Cognon C, Pradeau D, Florent M, et al. Aluminum contamination of parenteral nutrition and aluminum loading in children on long-

term parenteral nutrition. Journal of Pediatric Gastroenterology and Nutrition. 2003;36(4):448-53.

[16] Gomez-Alonso C, Menendez-Rodriguez P, Virgos-Soriano M, Fernandez-Martin J, Fernandez-Coto M, Cannata-Andia J. Aluminum-induced osteogenesis in osteopenic rats with normal renal function. Calcified Tissue International. 1999;64(6):534-41.

[17] Johnson TL, Gaddini G, Branscum AJ, Olson DA, Caroline-Westerlind K, Turner RT, et al. Effects of Chronic Heavy Alcohol Consumption and Endurance Exercise on Cancellous and Cortical Bone Microarchitecture in Adult Male Rats. Alcoholism: Clinical and Experimental Research. 2014;38(5):1365-72.

[18] Eleftheriou KI, Rawal JS, James LE, Payne JR, Loosemore M, Pennell DJ, et al. Bone structure and geometry in young men: the influence of smoking, alcohol intake and physical activity. Bone. 2013;52(1):17-26.

[19] Emaus N, Wilsgaard T, Ahmed LA. Impacts of Body Mass Index, Physical Activity, and Smoking on Femoral Bone Loss. The Tromsø Study. Journal of Bone and Mineral Research. 2014;29(9):2080-9.

[20] De Jong WU, de Jong PA, Vliegenthart R, Isgum I, Lammers JWJ, Oudkerk M, et al. Association of COPD and smoking status with bone density and vertebral fractures in male lung cancer screening participants. Journal of Bone and Mineral Research. 2014;29(10):2224-9.

[21] Callréus M, McGuigan F, Åkesson K. Adverse Effects of Smoking on Peak Bone Mass May Be Attenuated by Higher Body Mass Index in Young Female Smokers. Calcified Tissue International. 2013;93(6):517-25.

[22] Little RD, Folz C, Manning SP, Swain PM, Zhao S-C, Eustace B, et al. A mutation in the LDL receptor–related protein 5 gene results in the autosomal dominant high-bone-mass trait. The American Journal of Human Genetics. 2002;70(1):11-9.

[23] Boyden LM, Mao J, Belsky J, Mitzner L, Farhi A, Mitnick MA, et al. High bone density due to a mutation in LDL-receptor–related protein 5. New England Journal of Medicine. 2002;346(20):1513-21.

[24] Hoang BH, Kubo T, Healey JH, Sowers R, Mazza B, Yang R, et al. Expression of LDL receptor-related protein 5 (LRP5) as a novel marker for disease progression in high-grade osteosarcoma. International Journal of Cancer. 2004;109(1):106-11.

[25] Gong Y, Slee RB, Fukai N, Rawadi G, Roman-Roman S, Reginato AM, et al. LDL receptor-related protein 5 (LRP5) affects bone accrual and eye development. Cell. 2001;107(4):513-23.

[26] Zhao L, Shim JW, Dodge TR, Robling AG, Yokota H. Inactivation of Lrp5 in osteocytes reduces Young's modulus and responsiveness to the mechanical loading. Bone. 2013;54(1):35-43.

[27] Xiong DH, Lei SF, Yang F, Wang L, Peng YM, Wang W, et al. Low-Density Lipoprotein Receptor-Related Protein 5 (LRP5) Gene Polymorphisms are Associated with Bone Mass in both Chinese and Whites. Journal of Bone and Mineral Research. 2007;22(3):385-93.

[28] Kiel DP, Ferrari SL, Cupples LA, Karasik D, Manen D, Imamovic A, et al. Genetic variation at the low-density lipoprotein receptor-related protein 5 (LRP5) locus modulates Wnt signaling and the relationship of physical activity with bone mineral density in men. Bone. 2007;40(3):587-96.

[29] Frost M, Andersen T, Gossiel F, Hansen S, Bollerslev J, van Hul W, et al. Levels of serotonin, sclerostin, bone turnover markers as well as bone density and microarchitecture in patients with high-bone-mass phenotype due to a mutation in Lrp5. Journal of Bone and Mineral Research. 2011;26(8):1721-8.

[30] Campos-Obando N, Oei L, Hoefsloot LH, Kiewiet RM, Klaver CC, Simon ME, et al. Osteoporotic Vertebral Fractures During Pregnancy: Be Aware of a Potential Underlying Genetic Cause. The Journal of Clinical Endocrinology & Metabolism. 2014;99(4):1107-11.

[31] Fahiminiya S, Majewski J, Roughley P, Roschger P, Klaushofer K, Rauch F. Whole-exome sequencing reveals a heterozygous LRP5 mutation in a 6-year-old boy with vertebral compression fractures and low trabecular bone density. Bone. 2013;57(1): 41-6.

[32] Leupin O, Piters E, Halleux C, Hu S, Kramer I, Morvan F, et al. Bone overgrowth-associated mutations in the LRP4 gene impair sclerostin facilitator function. Journal of Biological Chemistry. 2011;286(22):19489-500.

[33] Morrison NA, Qi JC, Tokita A, Kelly PJ, Crofts L, Nguyen TV, et al. Prediction of bone density from vitamin D receptor alleles. Nature. 1994;367(6460):284-7.

[34] Uysal AR, Sahin M, Gürsoy A, Güllü S. Vitamin D receptor gene polymorphism and osteoporosis in the Turkish population. Genetic testing. 2008;12(4):591-4.

[35] Li Y, Xi B, Li K, Wang C. Association between vitamin D receptor gene polymorphisms and bone mineral density in Chinese women. Molecular Biology Reports. 2012;39(5):5709-17.

[36] Pouresmaeili F, Jamshidi J, Azargashb E, Samangouee S. Association between vitamin D receptor gene BsmI polymorphism and bone mineral density in a population of 146 Iranian women. Cell Journal (Yakhteh). 2013;15(1):75.

[37] Kurt O, Yilmaz-Aydogan H, Uyar M, Isbir T, Seyhan MF, Can A. Evaluation of ERα and VDR gene polymorphisms in relation to bone mineral density in Turkish postmenopausal women. Molecular Biology Reports. 2012;39(6):6723-30.

[38] Mosaad YM, Hammad EM, Fawzy Z, Abdal Aal IA, Youssef HM, ElSaid TO, et al. Vitamin D receptor gene polymorphism as possible risk factor in rheumatoid arthritis and rheumatoid related osteoporosis. Human Immunology. 2014;75(5):452-61.

[39] Rass P, Pákozdi A, Lakatos P, Zilahi E, Sipka S, Szegedi G, et al. Vitamin D receptor gene polymorphism in rheumatoid arthritis and associated osteoporosis. Rheumatology International. 2006;26(11):964-71.

[40] Jin H, Evangelou E, Ioannidis J, Ralston S. Polymorphisms in the 5′ flank of COL1A1 gene and osteoporosis: meta-analysis of published studies. Osteoporosis International. 2011;22(3):911-21.

[41] Wenstrup RJ, Lever LW, Phillips CL, Quarles LD. Mutations in the COL1A2 gene of type I collagen that result in nonlethal forms of osteogenesis imperfecta. American Journal of Medical Genetics. 1993;45(2):228-32.

[42] Spotila LD, Constantinou CD, Sereda L, Ganguly A, Riggs BL, Prockop DJ. Mutation in a gene for type I procollagen (COL1A2) in a woman with postmenopausal osteoporosis: evidence for phenotypic and genotypic overlap with mild osteogenesis imperfecta. Proceedings of the National Academy of Sciences. 1991;88(12):5423-7.

[43] Kurt-Sirin O, Yilmaz-Aydogan H, Uyar M, Seyhan M-F, Isbir T, Can A. Combined effects of collagen type I alpha1 (COL1A1) Sp1 polymorphism and osteoporosis risk factors on bone mineral density in Turkish postmenopausal women. Gene. 2014;540(2):226-31.

[44] Macdonald HM, McGuigan FA, New SA, Campbell MK, Golden MH, Ralston SH, et al. COL1A1 Sp1 polymorphism predicts perimenopausal and early postmenopausal spinal bone loss. Journal of Bone and Mineral Research. 2001;16(9):1634-41.

[45] Bernad M, Martinez M, Escalona M, Gonzalez M, Gonzalez C, Garces M, et al. Polymorphism in the type I collagen (COLIA1) gene and risk of fractures in postmenopausal women. Bone. 2002;30(1):223-8.

[46] Ralston SH, Uitterlinden AG, Brandi ML, Balcells S, Langdahl BL, Lips P, et al. Large-scale evidence for the effect of the COLIA1 Sp1 polymorphism on osteoporosis outcomes: the GENOMOS study. PLoS Medicine. 2006;3(4):e90.

[47] Lindberg MK, Weihua Z, Andersson N, Movérare S, Gao H, Vidal O, et al. Estrogen receptor specificity for the effects of estrogen in ovariectomized mice. Journal of Endocrinology. 2002;174(2):167-78.

[48] Turner RT. Mice, estrogen, and postmenopausal osteoporosis. Journal of Bone and Mineral Research. 1999;14(2):187-91.

[49] Korach KS. Insights from the study of animals lacking functional estrogen receptor. Science. 1994;266(5190):1524-7.

[50] Smith EP, Boyd J, Frank GR, Takahashi H, Cohen RM, Specker B, et al. Estrogen resistance caused by a mutation in the estrogen -receptor gene in a man. New England Journal of Medicine. 1994;331(16):1056-61.

[51] Ohlsson C, Engdahl C, Börjesson AE, Windahl SH, Studer E, Westberg L, et al. Estrogen receptor-α expression in neuronal cells affects bone mass. Proceedings of the National Academy of Sciences. 2012;109(3):983-8.

[52] Kondoh S, Inoue K, Igarashi K, Sugizaki H, Shirode-Fukuda Y, Inoue E, et al. Estrogen receptor α in osteocytes regulates trabecular bone formation in female mice. Bone. 2014;60:68-77.

[53] Guo Y, Wang J-T, Liu H, Li M, Yang T-L, Zhang X-W, et al. Are bone mineral density loci associated with hip osteoporotic fractures? A validation study on previously reported genome-wide association loci in a Chinese population. Genetics and molecular research: GMR. 2012;11(1):202.

[54] Canto-Cetina T, Polanco Reyes L, González Herrera L, Rojano-Mejía D, Coral-Vázquez RM, Coronel A, et al. Polymorphism of LRP5, but not of TNFRSF11B, is associated with a decrease in bone mineral density in postmenopausal maya-mestizo women. American Journal of Human Biology. 2013;25(6):713-8.

[55] van Meurs JB, Trikalinos TA, Ralston SH, Balcells S, Brandi ML, Brixen K, et al. Large-scale analysis of association between LRP5 and LRP6 variants and osteoporosis. Jama. 2008;299(11):1277-90.

[56] Zmuda JM. Identification of Osteoporosis Risk Genes: The Tip of the Iceberg. Annals of internal medicine. 2009;151(8):581-2.

[57] Agueda L, Urreizti R, Bustamante M, Jurado S, Garcia-Giralt N, Díez-Pérez A, et al. Analysis of three functional polymorphisms in relation to osteoporosis phenotypes: replication in a Spanish cohort. Calcified Tissue International. 2010;87(1):14-24.

[58] Kumar J, Swanberg M, McGuigan F, Callreus M, Gerdhem P, Åkesson K. LRP4 association to bone properties and fracture and interaction with genes in the Wnt-and BMP signaling pathways. Bone. 2011;49(3):343-8.

[59] Boudin E, Steenackers E, Freitas FD, Nielsen TL, Andersen M, Brixen K, et al. A common LRP4 haplotype is associated with bone mineral density and hip geometry in men – Data from the Odense Androgen Study (OAS). Bone. 2013;53(2):414-20.

[60] Tang PL, Cheung CL, Sham PC, McClurg P, Lee B, Chan SY, et al. Genome-Wide Haplotype Association Mapping in Mice Identifies a Genetic Variant in CER1 Associated With BMD and Fracture in Southern Chinese Women. Journal of Bone and Mineral Research. 2009;24(6):1013-21.

[61] Xiong D-H, Liu X-G, Guo Y-F, Tan L-J, Wang L, Sha B-Y, et al. Genome-wide Association and Follow-Up Replication Studies Identified ADAMTS18 and TGFBR3 as

Bone Mass Candidate Genes in Different Ethnic Groups. The American Journal of Human Genetics. 2009;84(3):388-98.

[62] Kuipers A, Zhang Y, Cauley JA, Nestlerode CS, Chu Y, Bunker CH, et al. Association of a high mobility group gene (HMGA2) variant with bone mineral density. Bone. 2009;45(2):295-300.

[63] Chen XD, Xiao P, Lei SF, Liu YZ, Guo YF, Deng FY, et al. Gene expression profiling in monocytes and SNP association suggest the importance of the STAT1 gene for osteoporosis in both Chinese and Caucasians. Journal of Bone and Mineral Research. 2010;25(2):339-55.

[64] Guo Y, Tan L-J, Lei S-F, Yang T-L, Chen X-D, Zhang F, et al. Genome-wide association study identifies ALDH7A1 as a novel susceptibility gene for osteoporosis. PLoS genetics. 2010;6(1):e1000806.

[65] Guo Y, Zhang LS, Yang TL, Tian Q, Xiong DH, Pei YF, et al. IL21R and PTH may underlie variation of femoral neck bone mineral density as revealed by a genome-wide association study. Journal of Bone and Mineral Research. 2010;25(5):1042-8.

[66] Koller DL, Ichikawa S, Lai D, Padgett LR, Doheny KF, Pugh E, et al. Genome-wide association study of bone mineral density in premenopausal European-American women and replication in African-American women. The Journal of Clinical Endocrinology & Metabolism. 2010;95(4):1802-9.

[67] Rivadeneira F, Styrkársdottir U, Estrada K, Halldórsson BV, Hsu YH, Richards JB, et al. Twenty bone-mineral-density loci identified by large-scale meta-analysis of genome-wide association studies. Nat Genet. 2009;41(11):1199-206.

[68] Richards JB1, Kavvoura FK, Rivadeneira F, Styrkársdóttir U, Estrada K, Halldórsson BV, et al. Collaborative meta-analysis: associations of 150 candidate genes with osteoporosis and osteoporotic fracture. Ann. Intern. Med. 2009;20;151(8):528-37.

[69] Kung AW1, Xiao SM, Cherny S, Li GH, Gao Y, Tso G, et al. Association of JAG1 with bone mineral density and osteoporotic fractures: a genome-wide association study and follow-up replication studies. Am. J. Hum. Genet. 2010;86(2):229-39.

[70] Hsu YH, Zillikens MC, Wilson SG, Farber CR, Demissie S, Soranzo N, et al. An integration of genome-wide association study and gene expression profiling to prioritize the discovery of novel susceptibility Loci for osteoporosis-related traits. PLoS Genet. 2010;6(6):e1000977.

[71] Cheung CL, Sham PC, Xiao SM, Bow CH, Kung AW. Meta-analysis of gene-based genome-wide association studies of bone mineral density in Chinese and European subjects. Osteoporos. Int. 2012;23(1):131-42.

[72] Estrada K, Styrkarsdottir U, Evangelou E, Hsu YH, Duncan EL, Ntzani EE, et al. Genome-wide meta-analysis identifies 56 bone mineral density loci and reveals 14 loci associated with risk of fracture. Nat. Genet. 2012;44(5):491-501.

[73] Zhang L, Choi HJ, Estrada K, Leo PJ, Li J, Pei YF, et al. Multistage genome-wide association meta-analyses identified two new loci for bone mineral density. Hum. Mol. Genet. 2014;23(7):1923-33.

[74] Iafrate AJ, Feuk L, Rivera MN, Listewnik ML, Donahoe PK, Qi Y, et al. Detection of large-scale variation in the human genome. Nature Genetics. 2004;36(9):949-51.

[75] Sebat J, Lakshmi B, Troge J, Alexander J, Young J, Lundin P, et al. Large-scale copy number polymorphism in the human genome. Science. 2004;305(5683):525-8.

[76] Yang T-L, Chen X-D, Guo Y, Lei S-F, Wang J-T, Zhou Q, et al. Genome-wide Copy-Number-Variation Study Identified a Susceptibility Gene, UGT2B17, for Osteoporosis. The American Journal of Human Genetics. 2008;83(6):663-74.

[77] Deng F-Y, Zhao L-J, Pei Y-F, Sha B-Y, Liu X-G, Yan H, et al. Genome-wide copy number variation association study suggested VPS13B gene for osteoporosis in Caucasians. Osteoporosis International. 2010;21(4):579-87.

[78] Oei L, Hsu Y-H, Styrkarsdottir U, Eussen BH, de Klein A, Peters MJ, et al. A genome-wide copy number association study of osteoporotic fractures points to the 6p25. 1 locus. Journal of Medical Genetics. 2014;51(2):122-31.

[79] Ran S, Liu Y-J, Zhang L, Pei Y, Yang T-L, Hai R, et al. Genome-Wide Association Study Identified Copy Number Variants Important for Appendicular Lean Mass. PloS One. 2014;9(3):e89776.

Chapter 4

Homocysteine and Leptin in the Pathogenesis of Osteoporosis — Evidences, Conflicts and Expectations

Mukhtiar Baig, Saba Tariq and Sundus Tariq

Additional information is available at the end of the chapter

http://dx.doi.org/10.5772/59869

1. Introduction

1.1. Homocysteine and leptin in the pathogenesis of osteoporosis: evidences, conflicts and expectations

1.1.1. Osteoporosis

Osteoporosis is a metabolic bone problem, also recognized as "the silent thief" because there is slow bone loss, generally occurs over the years, and without any symptoms until the bone becomes so brittle that suddenly fracture occurs. Osteoporosis is the most common disorder related to age [1]. It is a leading cause of fractures in old age: causing pain, affliction, hospitalization, financial burden, poor life quality leading to early death [2]. Osteoporosis is usually considered a normal part of the ageing process and an unavoidable consequence of growing older. However, osteoporosis is a detectable, preventable, and treatable disease.

1.1.2. Types of osteoporosis

Two types have been identified

- Primary osteoporosis.
  - **Type I** also called postmenopausal osteoporosis, occurs after menopause when the estrogen levels drop in the body. It typically involves the trabecular bone.
  - **Type II** also called senile osteoporosis, takes place after 70 years of age, involving both trabecular and cortical bone.
- Secondary osteoporosis.
  - It is due to the effect of medications like steroids or certain medical conditions.

1.1.3. Epidemiology

In postmenopausal females, osteoporosis has an enormous social and economic burden. With increasing age, the risk of osteoporotic fractures increases. There are about two million cases of fractures in the USA per year and out of them, there are about three hundred thousand hip fractures. The fractures and resultant health consequences have led to mortality rate up to 24% in women [3].

International osteoporosis foundation has estimated that globally osteoporosis affects one in three women and one in eight men above 50 years of age [4].

1.1.4. Pathogenesis

Osteoporosis develops when there is imbalance between the processes of bone resorption and bone formation. Osteoclasts (bone resorbing cells) eradicate bone by acidification and proteolytic digestion and osteoblasts (bone forming cells) secrete osteoid into the resorption cavity [5]. The normal cycle of bone turnover is needed for bone and maintenance of proper bodily functions. Each year 10 to 30% of the skeleton is remodeled in this way, and many hormones and chemical factors regulate this process and any change in these factors can manipulate the progress of osteoporosis. These influencing factors are estrogen, vitamin D, leptin, homocysteine, parathyroid hormone, testosterone, and blood factors involved in cell growth [6].

The bone turnover is perfectly balanced until the age of forty years. Nevertheless, old age, many diseases and medicines can disturb the balance, ultimately the breakdown process exceeds the bone formation, and as a result, trabecular plates of bone are destroyed causing weakness of the structure of bone with greatly reduced bone mass. Bone strength is a sign of the integration of bone quality (rate of bone remodeling, trabecular connectivity, degree of mineralization, and damage accumulation) and bone mineral density (BMD) [7]. There is doubling in the bone remodeling rate at menopause, becomes triple within 13 years of development of menopause and remains high till the development of osteoporosis. In osteoporosis, the trabecular bone loss is more as compared to cortical bone (50% as compared to 5%) and it occurs more swiftly in first 3-4 years after menopause [6].

1.1.5. Risk factors

It is a multifactorial disease including both modifiable and non-modifiable risk factors. Numerous factors are involved and augment the risk of developing osteoporosis [8-10].

- Non-modifiable risk factors
  - Increasing age
  - Female gender
  - Caucasian and Asian women and men
  - Small, thin-boned women
  - Maternal history of osteoporotic fracture
  - Deficiency of estrogen

http://dx.doi.org/10.5772/59869

- Modifiable risk factors
  - Smoking
  - Excessive alcohol consumption
  - Sedentary lifestyle over many years
  - Diet deficient in calcium
  - Insufficient exposure to sunlight, resulting in vitamin D deficiency
  - Hyperhomocysteinemia
  - Leptin

1.1.6. Homocysteine

Homocysteine (Hcy) is produced from the methionine metabolism, it is a sulfur-containing, nonproteinogenic amino acid (figure 1) [11]. Methionine, itself is a sulfur containing amino acid obtained from proteins of animal origin. It is metabolized in the body by either remethylation or transsulfuration pathway as shown in the figure 2. Both genetic (methylene tetrahydrofolate reductase or cystathionine β synthase polymorphisms) and environmental (age, renal function, B vitamins status) factors affect the plasma homocysteine concentration [12].

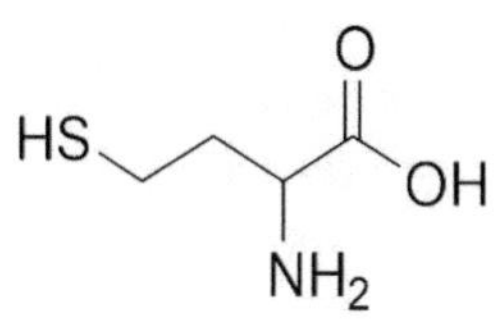

Figure 1. Structure of Homocysteine

2. Hcy and bone metabolism

Hyperhomocysteinemia (HHcy) is the elevated levels of total plasma Hcy. Generally, the Hcy level <15 μmol/L is considered normal but an increased plasma Hcy level (>15 μmol/L) is common in about 30–50% of elderly people (>60 years)[13]. There are multifactorial contributing factors like, a combination of genetic and environmental factors, lifestyle, diet, and hormonal factors might play a key role [14]. In addition, of being a known potent thrombogenic compound, [15] it has been proposed as a new risk factor for primary osteoporosis [16-18]. Like osteoporosis, HHcy is a frequent age related issue in aged people [19-20]. In old age, deficiency of vitamin B-12 and folate is common, and the prevalence of both vitamin deficiencies increases with age. Deficiency of either folate or vitamin B-12 results in increased tHcy levels because vit B12 acts as a cofactor for methionine synthase, the enzyme that remethylates homocysteine to methionine by using 5methyltetrahydrofolate as a methyl donor [20].

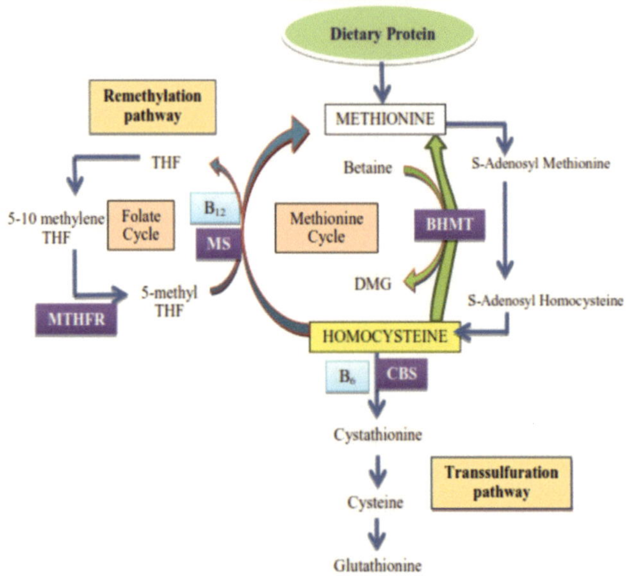

BHMT: betaine-homocysteine methyltransferase **DMG:** dimethylglycine **vitamin B6:** pyridoxyl phosphate **CBS:** cystathionine beta-synthase **vitamin B12:** cobalamine **MS:** methionine synthase **THF:** tetrahydrofolate **MTHFR:** 5,10-methylenetetrahydrofolate-reductase

Figure 2. Homocysteine metabolism

Ozdem et al., (2007) reported that experimental hyperhomocysteinemia disturbs bone metabolism in rats. They found that rats fed with a methionine-enriched diet had increased bone resorption markers (hydroxyproline & N-terminal collagen I telopeptides) and decreased bone formation marker (osteocalcin) [21]. Additionally, chronic HHcy may take part an imperative role in the development of arterial and venous thrombosis, senile osteoporosis, presbyopia and cognitive decline. These diseases are usually common in elderly [22]. An inverse correlation of total homocysteine (tHcy) concentrations with BMD has been documented by several reports, especially in postmenopausal women, and HHcy has been labeled as a modifiable risk factor for osteoporotic hip fracture [16-17, 23-26], while several other studies could not establish any correlation [27-29]. Similarly, an Italian study showed an inverse association of plasma concentration of tHcy with BMD of the total femur in post-menopausal women and the study concluded that it is independent of other recognized reasons of bone mineral loss, such as reduced BMI and old age [30]. Recently, in Pakistan, we investigated correlation of serum Hcy with BMD in postmenopausal osteoporotic females but could not find any correlation [31]. It has been reported that increased Hcy levels, decreased vitamin B12, and folate status have been related with reduced BMD and increased fracture risk and thus serum Hcy level can be used as an indicator of such micronutrient insufficiencies [16-17, 25, 27].

Herrmann et al., (2007) provided the first evidence regarding effects of chronic HHcy on bone quality in rats. In this study, healthy adult rats displayed reduction in bone strength in cancellous bone as reflected by biomechanical testing and histomorphometry, after 3 months of HHcy. The study did not explain the main mechanism behind this result [32]. Few mechanistic studies recommended that Hcy excites osteoclasts and causes disproportion between osteoclasts and osteoblasts in support of the osteoclasts, which are the main bone resorbing cells [33-36]. Furthermore, it appears that a number of extracellular mechanisms are also implicated. A study exhibited a reduced level of enzymatic cross-links in the bones of hyperhomocysteinemic female fracture patients that indicates impaired collagen cross-linking [37]. A study reported that in hyperhomocysteinemic animals, Hcy is deposited in bone tissue that causes considerable bone loss and consequently decreased bone strength [38].

3. Hcy and bone interaction: conflicts and evidences

During last few years, abundant literature has been published about the interaction of HHcy and bone. Up till now, several mechanisms have been proposed about the involvement of Hcy in bone pathology. HHcy is an emerging, but still non established, modifiable risk factor for osteoporotic fractures [39].

An elevated level of Hcy has been proposed as a new threat for primary osteoporosis [16-17]. Tyagi et al., 2011 in their study concluded that Hcy may cause reduced blood flow in bone as it stimulates the atherogenic process, promotes platelet adhesion and has also been recognized as a potent thrombogenic compound that might contribute to compromised bone biomechanical properties [40].

A prospective population-based study, reported that the highest quartile of tHcy was related with a two-fold augmented risk of fracture, and the relationship was continuous and there was 30% increased fracture risk with each standard deviation raise in tHcy [17]. Recently, a study by Enneman (2014) reported inverse correlation of plasma homocysteine levels with BMD [41].

In the early years of Hcy and bone research, it seemed that Hcy directly affects biomechanical properties because deposition of Hcy in bone coupled with a decrease in cancellous bone. A study suggested that deficiency of B12, folate and vitamin B6 elevates the plasma level of tHcy [35]. Another study found that the interaction of tHcy molecule with protein (collagen) in bone matrix takes place through thiol group and an amino group. This study also demonstrated that bone strength is reduced because most of the tHcy (65%) attaches with collagen [38].

A study proposed four mechanisms by which modification in bone remodeling takes place by tHcy: (i) enhancement in osteoclastic activity, (ii) reduction in osteoblastic activity, (iii) reduction in blood flow in bone, (iv) direct interaction of Hcy and bone matrix [42].

A study illustrated that tHcy inhibits lysyl oxidase, thus interferes with post-translational changes of collagen and this leads to decrease in bone quality [43]. The tHcy stimulated interleukin-6 (IL-6) production in osteoblasts, affects metabolism of bone by osteoclast. Janus kinase 2 (JAK2), DNA (cytosine-5) – methyltransferase 1 (DNMT1) stimulate IL-6, which affects bone matrix formation [44]. A study documented that the skeleton and muscles movements reduce tHcy level and this link was not dependent on vitamin supplements, vegetables and fruits intake. Thus, it was suggested that levels of tHcy are also mainly affected by physical activity, though, nutritional condition also contribute significantly [16]. Thus, it seems that, regular exercise may decrease the Hcy level in HHcy individuals while it may help in maintaining Hcy level in normal subjects.

A study observed that the maximum tertile of tHcy was related with a higher hip BMD loss over 4 years (-2.8%) compared to middle (-1.6%) and lowest tertiles (-1.2%) in elderly women (age ranges from 70 to 85 years). It was stated that the incidence and prevalence of fractures were not affected by elevated tHcy levels, but the augmented tHcy level is related with considerable hipbone loss in aged subject [45].

No association of fracture risk with tHcy in the highest quartile was shown in a study after adjustment for age but without adjustment of age risk was higher. They described that tHcy level could be modulated by nutritional conditions, renal failure and physical activity [46]. An animal study demonstrated that HHcy causes impairment in fracture repair. In their study, a closed femoral fracture was induced in mice after feeding them Hcy for 3 weeks, and biomechanical parameters were monitored after 4 weeks of healing. They found that hyperhomocysteinemic rats with fracture have reduced bending rigidity of femora and smaller callus diameter with no change in tissue composition and consequently it impaired fracture repair and reduced bone quality [47].

First clinical evidence about the relationship of HHcy and fracture risk came from the longitudinal study in healthy participants of different age groups of both genders [48]. The results showed that HHcy levels are the independent risk factor for the future worsening of bone mass in premenopausal women and men. Conversely, they could not find same results in postmenopausal women (PMW). It was suggested that, even if a high serum tHcy level in postmenopausal women is not a factor related to the reduction in BMD, so it is likely that HHcy may be implicated in the fractures risk in PMW via some other method not involving BMD.

It is known that in the regulation of osteoblasts function, estrogen receptors play important role and this phenomenon is particularly important after menopause in women [49]. Aaron et al., (2009) probed the link of tHcy levels and methylation of estrogen receptor α. Their data pointed out that tHcy can support hypermethylation of promoter A region, by this means decreases transcription of estrogen receptor α mRNA. It was anticipated that in the pathogenesis of postmenopausal osteoporosis it could be a probable mechanism. Therefore, an estrogen receptor mediated role of tHcy may cause worsening in biomechanical bone characteristics. Additionally, higher levels of Hcy lead to down regulation of estrogen receptor transcription in bone and other useful osteogenic effects turn out to be down regulated [50].

A study tried to devise some likely therapeutic options for reducing increased plasma levels of tHcy that may cause damaging effect on bone. They used strontium ranelate 2 g/day to lessen increased plasma levels of tHcy because such material found to extensively reduce tHcy concentrations in osteoporotic women and was suggested to be employed as a mean to lessen fracture risk by reducing tHcy levels [51]. Strontium ranelate was selected because of its recognized positive outcome of lessening resorption of bone and supporting bone construction. It is not unlikely that decrease in levels of tHcy is accountable for permitting the recognized effects of strontium ranelate to happen [52].

It is suggested that if changed bone biomechanical characteristics are result of increased Hcy and hormone replacement therapy (HRT) is recognized to ameliorate quality of bone, it was assumed that HRT would ameliorate quality of bone by reducing tHcy concentration. But the researcher could not confirm this effect of HRT on Hcy in postmenopausal osteoporotic women [53].

A study in hip arthroplasty patients because of osteoarthritis, tried to investigate the link of serum tHcy levels with osteoarthritis. But this study could not establish any noteworthy association of tHcy levels with biomechanical or morphological bone characteristics as evaluated by histomorphometry and DEXA [54]. Bayhan et al., (2009) demonstrated that elevated tHcy levels appear to influence bone quality and fracture risk, but there have been no distinguishing alterations in bone density [51].

The Hcy impairs the cross-linking of collagen and for the solidity and potency of the collagen network, these cross-links are essential. Any meddling in cross-link formation would therefore, affect the quality of bone matrix, which in turn causes the fragility of bones due to defective collagen formation but would not affect BMD, which is the representative of bone mineralization only [37]. It was found in an animal study that elevated levels of Hcy for three months increase femoral neck fragility by 18% in methionine-fed rats, and two-fold in Hcy-fed rats. Lumbar spine and femoral neck also demonstrated reduce biomechanical characteristics, however, more in methionine- versus Hcy-fed rats [32].

Recently, a meta-analysis by Zhong et al., (2014) suggested that vitamin B12 and Hcy levels were considerably elevated in postmenopausal osteoporotic (PMOP) group compared to controls and these were linked with BMD in PMOP [55].

Bone component	Effect	Mechanism
Osteoblast	Decrease activity Increase activity	Reducing OPG and elevating RANKL production in osteoblast [58] Moderate stimulation of osteoblast activity but predominant effect on osteoclast [35]
Osteoclast	Increase activity	Shift the OPG:RANKL ratio in favour of elevated osteoclast activity and reduced bone quality by altering the redox regulatory system in the osteoblast [40, 58]
Bone matrix	Degradation	Reduction in bone blood flow [40] Activation and amplification in matrix metallo-proteinases through generation of ROS [59]. By inhibiting enzyme of collagen cross-linking (lysyl hydroxylase and lysyl oxidase) thus directly manipulate the stable bone matrix formation [44, 60].
Osteocalcin	Inhibit secretion	Suppress the expression of OC mRNA [61]
Osteopontin	Activated	By enhancing the expression of osteopontin mRNA (6).

OPG osteoprotegrin, **RANKL** receptor activator of nuclear factor-κB ligand, **Hcy** Homocysteine, **ROS** reactive oxygen species, **MAPK** Mitogen-activated protein kinases, **OC** osteocalcin **mRNA** messenger ribonucleic acid.

Table 1. Effect of Homocysteine on different Bone components

A meta-analysis provided a proof on homocysteine and fracture risk, displaying that HHcy augments the fracture risk [56]. A very important evidence of effect of HHcy on fracture risk was provided by another meta-analysis including more than ten thousand subjects, demonstrated 4% augmented risk of fracture by per μmol/L raise in Hcy level [57].

3.1. Expectations

In spite of substantial evidence that indicating the direct damaging role of HHcy on bone metabolism, the role of serum tHcy in bone loss is still unclear. HHcy can be reduced by vit B12, and folate therapy, so by designing randomized controlled trials (RCTs) of B-vitamins vs. placebo, it is quite likely to establish whether tHcy is a contributory risk factor for bone fracture or not [62].There are few RCTs available in literature but because of various reasons these are not up to the mark.

Based on evidences, provided in the literature, it seems that HHcy may have negative role in bone metabolism generally and in the process of osteoporosis particularly. However, more interventional studies are required to confirm the unfavorable role of HHcy, particularly in subjects who are at the risk of developing low bone mass. It is suggested that there is a need to develop several multicenter, well-designed trials on determining the effects of Hcy-lowering treatment on the prevention and/or management of osteoporosis. These longitudinal trials would determine the accurate nature of Hcy and bone interaction and that will establish the outcome of different bisphosphonate therapies on Hcy levels in treating osteoporosis.

4. Leptin

Adipose tissue is the largest endocrine organ in the human body; it serves considerable role in the energy homeostasis and several metabolic processes. It also has a multifaceted association with the bone. It is a general phenomenon that with increasing age the fat tissue in the bone marrow increased while the bone mass decreased. It is because both the osteoblast and adipocyte are developed from the same cell lineage the mesenchymal stromal cells (MSCs). The segregation tendency to preadipocytes or preosteoblasts is competitive and being inhibited by each other. Nevertheless, published literature advocates that through adipokines, adipose tissue have intricate effects on bone metabolism [63]. The family of adipokines, including leptin, adiponectin, chemerin, resistin, omentin, visfatin and vaspin, take part in several physiological, biochemical and pathological processes, including, the glucose and lipid oxidation, energy expenditure, immunity, reproduction, inflammation, and others. Because of growing evidences regarding interaction of adipokines and bone metabolism, the researchers are paying special attention to their relationship.

Leptin is a diverse 16 kDa peptide hormone, which belong to the family of helical cytokine with lengthy chain (figure 3) [64]. Leptin is an important member of adipokine family that helps in regulation of food intake, energy homeostasis, reproduction, metabolism, immune function, bone physiology, tissue remodeling, neuroendocrine function and others [65].

Research has shown that leptin plays significant role in the regulation of body weight and BMD. Experimental evidence in mice showed that they appeared obese and have increased bone density when they were congenitally absent in leptin (ob/ob), indicating that leptin has a role in loss of bone density as well as fatty tissue [66].

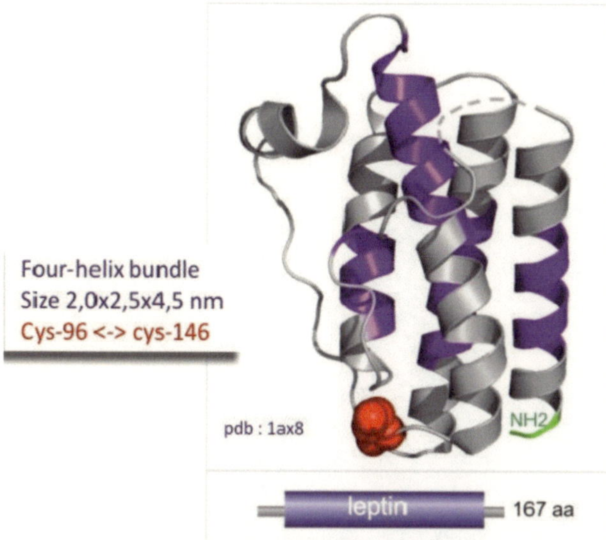

Figure 3. Leptin structure [64]

In a study, leptin replacement demonstrated the improvement of abnormalities in ob/ob mice in the form of decreasing food intake, energy loss, and temperature of body, infertility and immune function [67]. Since then, the knowledge which has been obtained from various studies indicating that leptin is not only important in control of body weight but also play imperative role in angiogenesis, hematopoiesis, blood pressure, immune function, lymphoid organ homeostasis, T lymphocyte systems, fertility, and bone formation [68].

Leptin is produced primarily from adipocytes according to adipose tissues quantity in the body. Brown fat tissue, stomach, placenta, ovary, bone marrow, liver, pituitary and mammary epithelial cells also secrete leptin [69]. Researchers observed that leptin is encoded by ob gene (LEP) (ob - obese and LEP - Leptin), according to the name that was first proposed, 'leptos', derived from the Greek word meaning thin, as ob protein is considered to be one of the molecules that regulates energy balance in mice [70].

4.1. Leptin receptor

Leptin's receptors were first isolated by cloning from mouse choroid plexus, these receptors belong to the cytokine family. There are six leptin receptors, which are divided into secretory (ob-Re), long (ob-Rb), and short forms (four short form receptors) [71-72]. The molecular receptor structure of the leptin and helical cytokine (class I) is similar. These homodimer receptors are able to activate the Janus kinase (JAK), and JAK is capable of starting as an activator of STAT – signal transducer and activator of transcription (Figure 4) [73]. Leptin signals through the activator system of JAK transcription, are associated with the form obRb (isoform long form) that would alter the expression of hypothalamic neuropeptides [74-75]. The ob-Rb is found in high levels in the hypothalamic nuclei [71] and its activity helps in mediating signal transduction by leptin in the hypothalamus, while the other leptin receptor activity (short form) is not strong enough in the functioning of leptin [72].

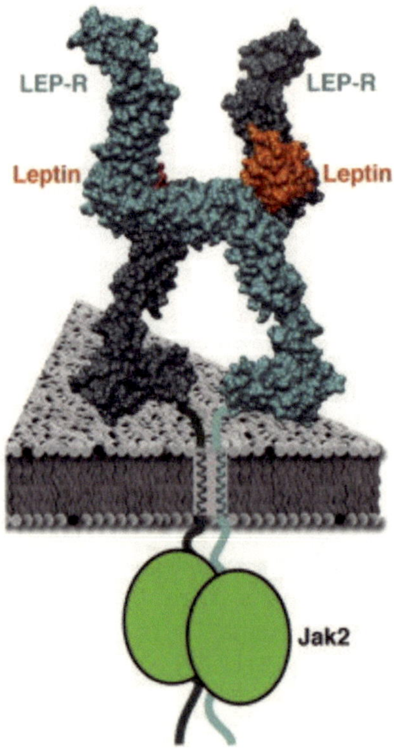

Figure 4. Leptin receptor [73]

4.2. Leptin and bone interaction: conflicts and evidences

Bone mass has been said to be regulated by leptin. The interaction of leptin with bone is multifaceted, related with location of bone. It also depends on the fact that whether leptin has a direct action on osteoblasts through receptors or it acts indirectly through the hypothalamus, it has the ability to both stimulate and inhibit bone formation [76-79]. Reduction in serum leptin levels are linked with decreased intake of food that might results in reduction in formation of bone and growth especially in children and adolescence [80-81]. In mice, lack of leptin also causes loss of bone and increased adiposity in bone marrow [82]. Leptin's enhanced levels and bone mass are associated with each other in obesity [83]. Leptin instead of supporting adipocyte phenotype of bone marrow stromal cells (BMSCs) supports osteoblast demonstrated by in vitro studies [78, 84-85]. Similarly, in vitro studies have demonstrated that in ovariectomized rats there was reduction in bone loss and suspension of tail after leptin treatment [86-87].

A study in Caucasian woman demonstrated that serum leptin had an inverse relationship with BMD, another study observed a positive connection [88-89]. A large-scale study established that serum leptin has no association with BMD [90]. Similarly, in another study no relation established between leptin and BMD [91]. Furthermore, it was suggested that leptin might be a forecaster of BMD in females with low BMD [92]. Recently, in Pakistan, we investigated correlation of serum leptin with BMD in postmenopausal osteoporotic females but no relationship was found [31].

In vitro data shows that serum leptin supports the segregation and development of the osteoblast lineage cells and controls development of osteoclast [92-93]. Some clinical data have shown an inverse relationship between bone resorption markers and serum leptin concentrations in postmenopausal women [89, 94] while other found a negative relationship [95-96].

Recently, Scotece et al., (2014) described that leptin level could be a valuable risk marker for osteoporosis [97]. A study by Suh et al., (2013) found that changes in serum osteocalcin were linked with leptin levels. It seems that there is connection between adipose tissue and bone [98]. On the other hand, Mohiti-Ardekani et al., (2014) reported that there is no correlation of circulating leptin concentrations with BMD and bone biochemical markers including osteocalcin [99].

4.3. Indirect role of leptin in bone metabolism

Leptin has both direct and indirect effects on bone. Indirect mechanisms have been revealed by experimental studies in mutant rats and mice that cannot synthesize leptin or do not have receptors for it. Leptin is carried across the blood brain barrier (BBB) by special receptors, which are located on the endothelial cells, the obRa receptors. In the brain leptin binds with obRb receptors which are located in hypothalamus and activates them. Binding of leptin with its receptors stimulate the expression of a hypothalamic osteoblast inhibitory factor (HOBIF) that lowers the ability of osteoblast to make bone matrix [76-77, 100-101]. And because of this mechanism, obese ob (Lep)–/– mice, due to lack of leptin have an unusually elevated bone mass.

Leptin stimulates bone formation via beta-1-adrenergic receptors and stimulation of the somatotropin-IGF-1 system [102]. Leptin inhibits activity of osteo-catabolic neuropeptide Y (NPY) and stimulates activity of osteo-anabolic systems, such as cocain and amphetamine-regulating transcript, via hypothalamic relays [103]. Moreover, leptin suppresses bone formation through beta-2-adrenergic receptors located in bone and inhibits serotonin production in the brain that result in loss of trabecular bone formation [104].

4.4. Direct role of leptin in bone metabolism

This is achieved by directly inhibiting the BMSCs to generate osteoclast while stimulating them to differentiate into osteoblasts [84, 93]. The BMSCs can be discriminated mainly into adipocytes or osteoblast cell family. These adipocytes in bone marrow provide leptin, which is able to inhibit adipogenesis discrimination of BMSC. It can excite discrimination of osteoblasts [84] while another study have pointed out that extremely elevated level of leptin causes apoptosis of BMSCs. A study reported that human osteoblasts, can begin producing and secreting leptin in the delayed matrix-mineralizing stage or shifting to osteocytes [85]. Proliferation of cultured human osteoblasts is also stimulated with leptin and it causes human BMSCs to express collagen-I, osteocalcin & alkaline phosphatase, and matrix mineralization [84,105]. These in vitro studies demonstrated that effects of leptin are dual in the microenvironment of bone and it also depends on presence of the leptin levels locally.

In the last decade, researchers proposed leptin to be a strong inhibitor of synthesis of bone because they could not find that osteoblast have long isoforms of the leptin receptors (ob-R) [76, 100]. In hypothalamus, and in many peripheral tissues expression of a large number of long isoform of ob-R have been confirmed [69].

Leptin receptors are also expressed by BMSCs, osteoblasts, osteoclasts and chondrocytes [84]. The signaling pathway in osteoblast, by which leptin acts, is osteoprotegerin (OPG)/RANKL (Receptor Activator for Nuclear factor κB Ligand). There was alteration found in the OPG/RANKL expression profile after treatment with leptin [93]. Burguera et al., (2001) have also established that bone loss in ovariectomized rats is reduced by elevating osteoprotegerin mRNA in osteoblasts [87].

For verifying the central effect, infusion of leptin was given into the brain and it was found that leptin also inhibits the bone formation through central nervous system. One important finding was that the lower doses inhibited the bone formation as compared to the doses which was essential for the loss of body weight [100-101]. It was observed in the experimental ob/ob mice that this central effect is due to activation of sympathetic part of autonomic nervous system. This activation of sympathetic system by leptin is very important in controlling energy homeostasis and numerous physiological functions [100].

In mice, food restriction decreased longitudinal growth and bone mass, but administration of leptin restored skeletal growth, in spite of low energy intake and raised serum osteocalcin, that is a bone formation marker [106].

In patients of hypothalamic amenorrhea, who have relative leptin deficiency, recombinant leptin treatment improves markers of bone formation [107]. It seems that leptin affects bone centrally through the sympathetic nervous system, which is a main downstream mediator [108]. Leptin deficiency seems to reduce adrenergic tone [109] and to influence the discharge of noradrenaline from sympathetic nerve fibers [110]. Noradrenaline binds to α -adrenergic receptors on osteoblasts and restrains formation of bone [108-109,111].

For observing direct and indirect or central and peripheral effects in vitro/in vivo, many researchers used supraphysiological doses of leptin in their studies [78,84,85,87], so it's difficult to draw accurate conclusion from these studies.

The mechanism of leptin function is highly intricate, because of the several receptor isoforms, localized expression and activation of leptin. Still, the role of leptin is not completely understood and the heterogeneity in its functions and its involvement in several body systems make its role challenging, particularly in the field of metabolism and endocrinology, and generally in medicine. Further studies are essentially needed for better understanding the role of leptin in several metabolic and non-metabolic functions that may also elucidate its role in health and disease and particularly in the pathophysiology of osteoporosis.

Bone component	Effect	Mechanism
Osteoblast	Increase directly	By inhibiting GSK-3β and thus promote differentiation of osteoblast and mineralization of primary cultures of VSMC [112]
Osteoblast	Decrease indirectly	By binding and activating obRb receptors, in hypothalamus. It stimulates the expression of a HOBIF that lowers the ability of osteoblast to make bone matrix [76-77, 100-101]
Osteoclast	Decrease	By inhibiting osteoclast generation by RANKL/RANK/OPG system [93]
Bone Matrix	Decrease	By inhibiting matrix mineralization. Endochondral ossification at the growth plate mediated by the leptin signaling[113]
Osteocalcin	Increase	By elevating osteoblast-specific osteocalcin release through a hypothalamic relay [114]
Osteopontin	Increase	By increasing up regulation of osteopontin by stimulating OPN mRNA and protein expression in these cells [115]

GSK glycogen synthase kinase, **VSMC** vascular smooth muscle cells **BBB** Blood Brain Barrier, **HOBIF** Hypothalamic osteoblast inhibitory factor, **OPG** osteoprotegrin, **RANKL** receptor activator of nuclear factor-κB ligand, **OPN** Osteopontin

Table 2. Effects of leptin on different Bone components

4.5. Expectations

Leptin replacement therapy in animals and humans has shown promising results, but, whether in postmenopausal osteoporotic patients, its use as a drug or drug target may give some therapeutic benefits; it's a basic question that is yet to be explored.

Therefore, in future, it could be expected that administration of some therapeutic agents that target the leptin secretion would contribute in decreasing the severity of the disease in postmenopausal women. Future studies may elucidate such agents and their role in alleviating progression and spread of osteoporosis. Serum leptin effects on bone metabolism are inconsistent and intricate, so there is still need to investigate the precise effects of leptin on bone by designing some clinical trials and longitudinal studies. Such studies would improve our understanding regarding the mechanisms underlying leptin role in bone metabolism and how it could be targeted particularly to treat osteoporosis or other bone disorders. Still, several venues need to be explored to explicate its undiscovered functions in human body especially, its role in terms of agonist and/or antagonist for the bone forming cells.

5. Conclusion

Evidences, shown by the results of several studies have clearly exhibited the role and involvement of leptin and Hcy in pathophysiology of osteoporosis at various levels but still their exact role, generally in bone metabolism and particularly in osteoporosis is not clear. We still need well designed experimental and clinical studies to validate the specific involvement of these two biochemical agents in bone pathophysiology or as a diagnostic & therapeutic markers, and also their precise involvement in osteoporosis and their synergistic, antagonists and/or agonists' influences on bone forming or destroying cells and other bone proteins.

It seems in future, leptin and Hcy could be the emerging therapies and new targets for treatment of osteoporosis. However, it would be too early to validate the role of Hcy and leptin in osteoporosis before addressing some important queries: like identifying their actual mechanism of action, site/s of their targets in the body for influencing bone metabolism, the effects of presently available anti-resorptive treatment on Hcy and leptin levels. Although, various studies have revealed mechanism of Hcy and leptin action, still further clarification regarding bone specific receptors, peripheral or central or both actions and their interaction with osteoporotic risk factors need to be investigated.

Numerous basic and clinical studies are available which are helping us to understand their role in health and diseases but still these are far from completion. Our future research should be focused on these important questions that whether bringing change in their level and/or activity may help us in preventing and treating osteoporosis, and interaction of Hcy and leptin with several other hormones and peptides and consequences of their increased/decreased levels at various tissues and organs level. Such questions require to be addressed for establishing their precise role in bone metabolism. Therefore, further studies are needed to reveal their character as novel therapeutic agents and/or targets.

6. Few key points

- Homocysteine (Hcy) and leptin are new risk factor for primary osteoporosis.
- Hcy interacts with bone by enhancing osteoclastic and reducing osteoblastic activity, reducing bone blood supply and directly interacting with bone matrix.
- Hcy level could be modulated by nutritional conditions, and physical activity.
- Each μmol/L raise in Hcy level augments 4% fracture risk.
- Serum leptin supports the segregation and development of the osteoblast lineage cells and control development of osteoclast.
- Leptin stimulates bone formation via beta-1-adrenergic receptors and stimulation of the somatotropin-IGF-1 system
- Leptin directly inhibits the BMSCs to generate osteoclast and stimulate them to differentiate into osteoblasts.

- BMSCs, osteoblasts, osteoclasts and chondrocytes have leptin receptors.
- The mechanism of leptin function is highly intricate, because of the several receptor isoforms, localized expression and activation of leptin.
- Leptin and Hcy role as diagnostic & therapeutic markers in osteoporosis needs further exploration.
- Further well-designed experimental and clinical studies are needed to validate the specific involvement of these two biochemical agents in bone pathophysiology.

Author details

Mukhtiar Baig[1], Saba Tariq[2] and Sundus Tariq[3]

*Address all correspondence to: drmukhtiarbaig@yahoo.com

1 Department of Clinical Biochemistry, Faculty of Medicine, Rabigh, King Abdulaziz University, Jeddah, KSA

2 Department of Pharmacology, University Medical & Dental College, The University of Faisalabad, Faisalabad, Pakistan

3 Department of Physiology, University Medical & Dental College, The University of Faisalabad, Faisalabad, Pakistan

References

[1] Lippuner K, Golder M, Greiner R. Epidemiology and direct medical costs of osteoporotic fractures in men and women in Switzerland. Osteoporosis International, 2005;16(2), S8-S17.

[2] Burge R, Dawson-Hughes B, Solomon DH, Wong JB, King A, Tosteson A. Incidence and economic burden of osteoporosis-related fractures in the United States, 2005–2025. J Bone Miner Res. 2007; 22: 465–75.

[3] LeBoff MS, Hawkes WG, Glowacki J, Yu-Yahiro J, Hurwitz S, Magaziner J. Vitamin D deficiency and post-fracture changes in lower extremity function and falls in women with hip fractures. Osteoporos Int 2008; 19: 1283–1290.

[4] IOF, International osteoporosis foundation. (2002). International osteoporosis foundation Annual Report 2002. [online] Available at: <http://www.iofbonehealth.org/download/osteofound/filemanager/publications/pdf/report_2002.pdf> [Accessed 24 June 2014].

[5] Manolagas SC. Birth and death of bone cells: basic regulatory mechanisms and implications for the pathogenesis and treatment of osteoporosis. Endocr Rev 2000; 21: 115–137.

[6] Cheung AM, Chaudhry R, Kapral M, Jackevicius C, Robinson G. Perimenopausal and postmenopausal health. BMC Womens Health 2004; 4: S1- S23.

[7] National institutes of health consensus development panel on osteoporosis, prevention, diagnosis and therapy. JAMA 2001; 285(6): 785–795.

[8] Servier. Causes of osteoporosis. [online] Available at: <http://www.servier.co.uk/disease-information/osteoporosis/causes-of-osteoporosis (2011). asp> [Accessed 20 June 2012].

[9] Sipos W, Pietschmann P, Rauner M, Kerschan-Schindl K. and Patsch J. Pathophysiology of osteoporosis. Wien. Med. Wochenschr., 2009;159: 230–234.

[10] Noale M, Maggi S, Crepaldi G. Osteoporosis among Italian women at risk: the OSTEOLAB study. J Nutr Health Aging 2012;16: 529-533.

[11] Selhub J. Homocysteine metabolism. Annu Rev Nutr 1999; 19: 217–246.

[12] Cattaneo M. Hyperhomocysteinemia, atherosclerosis and thrombosis. ThrombHaemost 1999; 81: 165–176.

[13] de Bree, NM, van der Put LI, Mennen L. et al. Prevalences of hyperhomocysteinemia, unfavorable cholesterol profile and hypertension in European populations. Eur J Clin Nutr 2005; 59(4): 480–488.

[14] Eussen SMP, De Groot PMG, Clarke R et al. Oral cyanocobalamin supplementation in older people with vitamin B 12 deficiency: a dose-finding trial. Arch Int Med 2005; 165(10): 1167-1172.

[15] Brattstrom LE, Hardebo JE, Hultberg BL. Moderate homocysteinemia possible risk factor for arteriosclerotic cerebrovascular disease. Stroke 1984; 15: 1012-1016.

[16] McLean RR, Jacques PF, Selhub J, Tucker KL, Samelson EJ, Broe KE, et al. Homocysteine as a predictive factor for hip fracture in older persons. N Engl J Med 2004; 351: 2042–2049.

[17] van Meurs JBJ, Dhonukshe-Rutten RAM, Pluijm SM, van der Klift M, de Jonge R, Lindemans J, et al. Homocysteine levels and the risk of osteoporotic fracture. N Engl J Med 2004; 350: 2033–2041.

[18] Hermann M, Schmidt PJ, Umanskaya N, wagner A, Taban-Shomal, widmann T, et al. The role of hyperhomocysteinemia as well as folate, vitamin B(6) and B(12) deficiencies in osteoporosis: a systematic review. Clin Chem. Lab Med 2007; 45: 1621–1632.

[19] Stranger O, Hermann W, Pietraik K et al., DACH-LIGA homocysteine (German, Austrian and Swisshomocysteine society): consensus paper on the rational clinical use of

homocysteine, folic acid and B-vitamins in cardiovascular and thrombotic diseases: guidelines and recommendations. Clin Chem Lab Med 2003; 41: 1392–1403.

[20] Clark R, Refsum H, Birks J et al. Screening for vitamin B 12 and folate deficiency in older persons.Am J Clin Nutr 2003;77: 1241–1247.

[21] Ozdem S, Samanci S, Tasatargil A, et al. Experimental hyperhomocysteinemia disturbs bone metabolism in rats. Scand J Clin Lab Invest. 2007; 67(7): 748–756.

[22] Krumdieck CL, Prince CW. Mechanisms of homocysteine toxicity on connective tissue: implications for the morbidity of aging. J Nutr 2000; 130: 365S–8S.

[23] Morris MS, Jacques PF, Selhub J. Relation between homocysteine and B-vitamin status indicators and bone mineral density in older Americans. Bone 2005; 37: 234–242.

[24] Refsum H, Nurk E, Smith D, Ueland PM, Gjesdal CG, Bjelland I, et al. The Hordal and Homocysteine Study: a community-based study of homocysteine, its determinants and associations with disease. J Nutr 2006; 136: 1731S–40S.

[25] Gjesdal CG, Vollset SE, Ueland PM, Refsum H, Drevon CA, Gjessing HK, et al. Plasma total homocysteine level and bone mineral density. The Hordaland Homocysteine Study. Arch Int Med 2006; 166: 88–94.

[26] LeBoff MS, Narweker R, LaCroix A, Wu LL, Jackson R, Lee J, et al. Homocysteine levels and risk of hip fracture in postmenopausal women. J Clin Endocrinol Metab 2009; 94: 1207–1213.

[27] Cagnacci A, Baldassari F, Rivolta G, Arangino S, Volpe A. Relation of homocysteine, folate and vitamin B12 to bone mineral density of postmenopausal women. Bone 2003; 33: 956–959.

[28] Bathum L, Von B, Hjelmborg J, Christiansen L, Skov MJ, Skytthe A, Christensen K. Evidence for an association of methylene tetrahydrofolatereductase polymorphism C677T and an increased risk of fractures: results from a population-based Danish twin study. Osteoporos Int. 2004; 15: 659–664.

[29] Sato Y, Iwamoto J, Kanoko T, Satoh K. Homocysteine as a predicitive factor for hip fracture in elderly women with Parkinson's disease. Am J Med 2005; 118: 1250–5.

[30] Bucciarelli P, Martini G, Martinelli I et al. The relationship between plasma homocysteine levels and bone mineral density in post-menopausal women. Eur J Int Med 2010; 21(4): 301–30.

[31] Tariq S, Tariq S, Alam SS, Baig M. Effect of Ibandronate treatment on serum homocysteine and leptin level in postmenopausal osteoporotic females. Osteoporosis International 2014, DOI: 10.1007/s00198-014-2909-9

[32] Herrmann M, Wildemann B, Claes L, Klohs S, Ohnmacht M, Taban-Shomal O, et al. Experimental hyperhomocysteinemia reduces bone quality in rats. Clin Chem 2007; 53: 1455–1461.

[33] Herrmann M, Widmann T, Colaianni G, Colucci S, Zallone A, Herrmann W. Increased osteoclast activity in the presence of increased homocysteine concentrations. Clin Chem 2005; 51: 2348–53.

[34] Koh JM, Lee YS, Kim YS, et al. Homocysteine enhances bone resorption by stimulation of osteoclast formation and activity through increased intracellular ROS generation. J Bone Miner Res 2006; 21: 1003–1011.

[35] Herrmann M, Umanskaya N, Wildemann B, et al. Stimulation of osteoblast activity by homocysteine. J Cell Mol Med 2008; 12: 1205–1210.

[36] Herrmann M, Umanskaya N, Wildemann B, et al. Accumulation of homocysteine by decreasing concentrations of folate, vitamin B12 and B6 does not influence the activity of human osteoblasts in vitro. Clin Chim Acta 2007; 384: 129–134.

[37] Saito M, Fujii K, Marumo K. Degree of mineralization-related collagen crosslinking in the femoral neck cancellous bone in cases of hip fracture and controls. Calcif Tissue Int 2006; 79: 160–168.

[38] Herrmann M, Tami A, Wildemann B, et al. Hyperhomocysteinemia induces a tissue specific accumulation of homocysteine in bone by collagen binding and adversely affects bone. Bone 2009; 44(3): 467–475.

[39] Dhonukshe-Rutten RA, Pluijm SM, de Groot LC, Lips P, Smit JH, van Staveren WA: Homocysteine and vitamin B12 status relate to bone turnover markers, broadband ultrasound attenuation, and fractures in healthy elderly people. J Bone Miner Res 2005, 20:921–929.

[40] Tyagi N, Vacek TP, Fleming JT, Vacek JC, Tyagi SC. Hyperhomocysteinemia decreases bone blood flow. Vasc Health Risk Manag 2011; 7: 31–35.

[41] Enneman WA, Swart MK, Zillikens CM, et al. The association between plasma homocysteine levels and bone quality and bone mineral density parameters in older persons. Bone 2014;63: 141–146

[42] Herrmann M, Widmann T, Herrmann W. Homocysteine – a newly recognised risk factor for osteoporosis. Clin Chem Lab Med 2005; 43: 1111–1117.

[43] Liu G, Nellaiappan K, Kagan HM. Irreversible inhibition of lysyl oxidase by homocysteinethiolactone and its selenium and oxygen analogues. Implications for homocystinuria. J Bio Chem 1997; 272: 32370–7.

[44] Thaler R, Agsten M, Spitzer S, Paschalis EP, Karlic H, Klaushofer K, et al. Homocysteine suppresses the expression of the collagen cross-linker lysyl oxidase involving IL-6, Fli1, and epigenetic DNA methylation. J Bio Chem 2011; 286: 5578–5588.

[45] Zhu K, Beilby J, Dick IM, Devine A, So o s M, Prince RL. The effects of homocysteine and MTHFR genotype on hip bone loss and fracture risk in elderly women. Osteoporos Int 2009; 20: 1183–1191.

[46] Perier MA, Gineyts E, Munoz F, Sornay-Rendu E, Delmas PD. Homocysteine and fracture risk in postmenopausal women: the OFELY study. Osteoporos Int 2007; 18: 1329–1336.

[47] Claes L, Schmalenbach J, Herrmann M, Olk UI, Garcia P, Histing T, et al. Hyperhomocysteinemia is associated with impaired fracture healing in mice. Calcif Tissue Int 2009; 85: 17–21.

[48] Kim BJ, Koh JM, Ahn SH et al., High serum total homocysteine levels accelerate hip bone loss in healthy pre-menopausal women and men. Bone 2013;52:56–62

[49] Levin ER. Plasma membrane estrogen receptors. Trends Endo crinol Metab 2009; 20: 477–482.

[50] Aaron W, Alexander A, Brugmann SA, Xu Y, Carre AL, Leucht P, et al. Estrogen/estrogen receptor α signaling in mouse posterofrontal cranial suture fusion. PLoS One 2009; 4: e7120.

[51] Bayhan I, Uygur D, Ugurlu N, Ozaksit G. Strontium ranelate decreases plasma homocysteine levels in postmenopausal osteoporotic women. Rheumatol Int 2009; 29: 263–266.

[52] Marie PJ, Ammann P, Boivin G, Rey C. Mechanisms of action and therapeutic potential of strontium in bone. Calcif Tissue Int 2001; 69: 121–129.

[53] Mijatovic V, van der Mooren MJ. Homocysteine in postmenopausal women and the importance of hormone replacement therapy. Clin Chem Lab Med 2001; 39: 764–767.

[54] Holstein JH, Herrmann M, Splett C, Herrmann W, Garcia P, Histing T, et al. Hyperhomocysteinemia is not associated with reduced bone quality in humans with hip osteoarthritis. Clin Chem Lab Med 2010; 48: 821–827.

[55] Zhang H, Tao X, Wu J. Association of homocysteine, vitamin B12, and folate with bone mineral density in postmenopausal women: a meta-analysis. Arch Gynecol Obstet 2014;289:1003–1009

[56] Yang J, Hu X, Zhang, Q, Cao H, Wang J, Liu B. Homocysteine level and risk of fracture: a meta-analysis and systematic review. Bone 2012; 51(3): 376–382.

[57] vanWijngaarden JP, Doets LE, SzczeciNska A, et al. Vitamin B12, folate, homocysteine, and bone health in adults and elderly people: A Systematic review with Meta-Analyses. J Nutr Metab (2013), http://dx.doi.org/10.1155/2013/486186.

[58] Vijayan V, Khandelwal M, Manglani K et al. Homocysteine alters the osteoprotegerin/RANKL system in the osteoblast to promote bone loss: pivotal role of the redox regulator forkhead O1. Free Radic Biol Med 2013;15;61C:72-84. doi: 0.1016/j.freeradbiomed.2013.03.004.

[59] Vacek TP, Kalani A, Voor MJ, Tyagi SC, Tyagi N. The role of homocysteine in bone remodeling. Clin Chem Lab Med 2013;51(3): 579–590. doi:10.1515/cclm-2012-0605.

[60] Thaler R, Spitzer S, Rumpler M, et al. Differential effects of homocysteine and beta aminopropionitrile on preosteoblastic MC3T3-E1 cells. Bone 2010;46(3):703-9. doi: 10.1016/j.bone.2009.10.038

[61] Sakamoto W, Isomura H, Fujie K. Homocysteine attenuates the expression of osteocalcin but enhances osteopontin in MC3T3-E1 preosteoblastic cells. Biochimica et Biophysica Acta 2005;1740:12 – 16

[62] Gommans J, Yi Q, Eikelboom JW, Hankey GJ, Chen C, Rodgers H.The effect of homocysteine-lowering with B-vitamins on osteoporotic fractures in patients with cerebrovascular disease: substudy of VITATOPS, a randomised placebo-controlled trial.BMC Geriatrics 2013; 13:88. doi:10.1186/1471-2318-13-88

[63] Liu Y, Song CY, Wu SS, Liang QH, Yuan LQ, & Liao E Y. Novel adipokines and bone metabolism. International journal of endocrinology, 2013, Article ID 895045, 9 pages. http://dx.doi.org/10.1155/2013/895045

[64] Homoeostasis regulation of food intake. Obesity project SV1632. http://www.cellbiol.net/ste/alpobesity2.php. [Accessed on 22 September, 2014]

[65] Stofkova A. Leptin and adiponectin: from energy and metabolic dysbalance to inflammation and autoimmunity. Endocr Regul 2009; 43(4): 157–168.

[66] Friedman JM, Halaas JL. Leptin and the regulation of body weight in mammals. Nature 1998; 395(6704): 763–70.

[67] Chehab FF, Lim ME, Rongue L. Correction of the sterility defect in homozygous obese female mice by treatment with the human recombinant leptin. Nat Genet 1996;12:318-320.

[68] Huang L, Li C. Leptin: a multifunctional hormone. Cell Res 2000; 10(2): 81–92.

[69] Zhang F, Chen Y, Heiman M, Dimarchi R. Leptin: structure, function and biology. Vitam Horm 2005; 71: 345–372.

[70] Zhang Y, Proenca R, Maffei M, Barone M, Leopold L, Friedman JM. Positional cloning of the mouse obese gene and its human homologue. Nature 1994; 372(6505): 425–432.

[71] Tartaglia LA, Dembski M, Weng X, Deng N, Culpepper J, Devos R, et al. Identification and expression cloning of a leptin receptor, OBR. Cell 1995; 83(7): 1263–1271.

[72] Hoggard N, Mercer JG, Rayner DV, Moar K, Trayhurn P, Williams LM. Localization of leptin receptor mRNA splice variants in murine peripheral tissues by RT-PCR and in situ hybridization. Biochem Biophys Res Commun 1997; 232(2): 383–387.

[73] Mancour VL, Daghestani HN, Dutta S, et al. Ligand- induced architecture of the leptin receptor signaling complex. Molecular Cell 2012; 48(4): 655–661.

[74] Bjorbaek C, Kahn BB. Leptin signaling in the central nervous system and the periphery. Recent ProgHorm Res 2004; 59: 305–331.

[75] Kelesidis T, Kelesidis I, Chou S, Mantzoros CS. Narrative review: the role of leptin in human physiology: emerging clinical applications. Ann Int Med 2010; 152(2): 93–100.

[76] Ducy P, Amling M, Takeda S, Priemel M, Schilling AF, Beil FT, et al. Leptin inhibits bone formation through a hypothalamic relay: A central control of bone mass. Cell 2000; 100: 197–207.

[77] Karsenty G. Leptin controls bone formation through a hypothalamic relay. Recent Prog Horm Res 2001; 56: 401–415.

[78] Cornish J, Callon KE, Bava U, Lin C, Naot D, Hill BL, et al. Leptin directly regulates bone cell function in vitro and reduces bone fragility in vivo. J Endocrinol 2002; 175: 405–415.

[79] Hamrick MW, Della-Fera MA, Choi YH, Hartzell D, Pennington C, Baile CA. Injections of leptin into rat ventromedial hypothalamus increase adipocyte apoptosis in peripheral fat and in bone marrow. Cell Tissue Res 2007; 327: 133–141.

[80] Chan JL, Mantzoros CS. Role of leptin in energy-deprivation states: Normal human physiology and clinical implications for hypothalamic amenorrhoea and anorexia nervosa. Lancet 2005; 366: 74–85.

[81] Hamrick MW. Leptin, bone mass, and the thrifty phenotype. J Bone Miner Res 2004; 19: 1607–1611.

[82] Hamrick MW, Pennington C, Newton D, Xie D, Isales C. Leptin deficiency produces contrasting phenotypes in bones of the limb and spine. Bone 2004; 34: 376–383.

[83] Goulding A, Taylor RW. Plasma leptin values in relation to bone mass and density and to dynamic biochemical markers of bone resorption and formation in postmenopausal women. Calcif Tissue Int 1998; 63: 456–458.

[84] Thomas T, Gori F, Khosla S, Jensen MD, Burguera B, Riggs BL. Leptin acts on human marrow stromal cells to enhance differentiation to osteoblasts and to inhibit differentiation to adipocytes. Endocrinology 1999; 140: 1630–1638.

[85] Reseland JE, Syversen U, Bakke I, Qvigstad G, Eide LG, Hjertner O, et al. Leptin is expressed in and secreted from primary cultures of human osteoblasts and promotes bone mineralization. J Bone Miner Res 2001; 16: 1426–1433.

[86] Martin A, de Vittoris R, David V, Moraes R, Begeot M, Lafage-Proust MH, et al. Leptin modulates both resorption and formation while preventing disuse induced bone loss in tail suspended female rats. Endocrinology 2005; 146: 3652–3659.

[87] Burguera B, Hofbauer LC, Thomas T, Gori F, Evans GL, Khosla S, et al. Leptin reduces ovariectomy-induced bone loss in rats. Endocrinology 2001; 142: 3546–3553.

[88] Kontogianni MD, Dafni UG, Routsias JG, Skopouli FN. Blood leptin and adiponectin as possible mediators of the relation between fat mass and BMD in perimenopausal women. J Bone Miner Res 2004; 19: 546–551.

[89] Blain H, Vuillemin A, Guillemin F, et al. Serum leptin level is a predictor of bone mineral density in postmenopausal women. J Clin Endocrinol Metab 2002; 87: 1030–1035.

[90] Ruhl CE, Everhart JE. Relationship of serum leptin concentration with bone mineral density in the United States population. J Bone Miner Res 2002; 17: 1896–1903.

[91] Wu N, Wang PQ, Li Hui, Wu PX, Sun QZ, Luo HX. Relationships between serum adiponectin, leptin concentrations and bone mineral density, and bone biochemical markers in Chinese women. Clinica Chimica Acta 2010; 411: 771–775.

[92] Gordeladze JO, Drevon CA, Syversen U, Reseland JE. Leptin stimulates human osteoblastic cell proliferation, de novo collagen synthesis, and mineralization: impact on differentiation markers, apoptosis, and osteoclastic signaling. J Cell Biochem 2002; 85: 825–836.

[93] Holloway WR, Collier FM, Aitken CJ, et al. Leptin inhibits osteoclast generation. J Bone Miner Res 2002; 17: 200–209.

[94] Cakmak A, Posaci C, Dogan E, Caliskan S, Guclu S, Altunyurt S. Raloxifene increases serum leptin levels in postmenopausal women: a prospective study. Am J Obstet Gynecol 2005; 193: 347–351.

[95] Yamauchi M, Sugimoto T, Yamaguchi T, et al. Plasma leptin concentrations are associated with bone mineral density and the presence of vertebral fractures in postmenopausal women. Clin Endocrinol (Oxf) 2001; 55: 341–347.

[96] Schett G, Kiechl S, Bonora E, et al. Serum leptin level and the risk of nontraumatic fracture. Am J Med 2004; 117: 952–956.

[97] Scotece M, Conde J, Vuolteenaho K et al. Adipokines as drug targets in joint and Bone disease. Drug Discovery Today 2014;19:241-258

[98] Suh H, Hwang I, Lee K, Kim K. Relationships between serum osteocalcin, leptin and the effect of weight loss by pharmacological treatment in healthy, nonsmoking Korean obese adults. Clinica Chimica Acta 2013; 418: 17–21.

[99] Mohiti-Ardekani J, Owlia MB, Soleymani-Salehabadi H, Mohiti A. Relationships between serum adipocyte hormones (adiponectin, leptin, resistin), bone mineral density and bone metabolic markers in osteoporosis patients. J Bone Miner Metab 2014; 32:400–404. DOI 10.1007/s00774-013-0511-4

[100] Ducy P, Schinke T, Karsenty G. The osteoblast: a sophisticated fibroblast under central surveillance. Science 2000; 289: 1501–1504.

[101] Amling M, Takeda S, Karsenty GA. Neuro(endo)crine regulation of bone remodeling. Bioessays 2000; 22: 970–975.

[102] Hamrick M W, Ferrari SL. Leptin and the sympathetic connection of fat to bone. Osteoporosis Intern 2008;19(7) 905-912.

[103] Kristensen P, Judge M E, Thim L., et al. Hypothalamic CART is a new anorectic peptide regulated by leptin. Nature 1998;393.6680: 72-76.

[104] Motyl KJ, Rosen CJ. Understanding leptin-dependent regulation of skeletal homeostasis. Biochemie 94: 2089-2096, 2012.

[105] Evans BAJ, Elford C, Gregory JW. Leptin control of bone metabolism; direct or indirect action? Bone 2001; 28:149.

[106] Gat-Yablonski G, Ben-Ari T, Shtaif B, et al. Leptin reverses the inhibitory effect of caloric restriction on longitudinal growth. Endocrinology 2004;145:343-350.

[107] Welt CK, Chan JL, Bullen J, et al. Recombinant human leptin in women with hypothalamic amenorrhea. N Engl J Med 2004;351:987-997.

[108] Lee NJ, Wong IP, Baldock PA, Herzog H. Leptin as an endocrine signal in bone. Curr Osteoporos Rep 2008;6:62-66.

[109] Elmquist JK, Maratos-Flier E, Saper CB, Flier JS. Unraveling the central nervous system pathways underlying responses to leptin. Nat Neurosci 1998;1:445-450.

[110] Elefteriou F, Ahn JD, Takeda S, et al Leptin regulation of bone resorption by the sympathetic nervous system and CART. Nature 2005;434:514-520.

[111] Jouanny P, Guillemin F, Kuntz C, Jeandel C, Pourel J. Environmental and genetic factors affecting bone mass. Similarity of bone density among members of healthy families. Arthritis Rheum 1995;38:61-67.

[112] Zeadin MG, Butcher MK, Shaughnessy SG, Werstuck GH. Leptin promotes osteoblast differentiation and mineralization of primary cultures of vascular smooth muscle cells by inhibiting glycogen synthase kinase (GSK)-3β. Biochem Biophys Res Commun 2012;425(4):924-930

[113] Kishida Y, Hirao M, Tamai N, et al. Leptin regulates chondrocyte differentiation and matrix maturation during endochondral ossification. Bone 2005;37(5): 607-621.

[114] Kalra SP, Dube MG, Iwaniec UT. Leptin increases osteoblast-specific osteocalcin release through a hypothalamic relay. Peptides 2009; 30(5):967-973.

[115] Sahai A, Malladi P, Pan X, Paul R et al. Obese and diabetic db/db mice develop marked liver fibrosis in a model of nonalcoholic steatohepatitis: role of short-form leptin receptors and osteopontin. American Journal of Physiology-Gastrointestinal and Liver Physiology 2004;287(5):G1035-G1043.

Chapter 5

Biological Effects of Skeletal Renin-Angiotensin System in Osteoporosis

Yan Zhang and Liang Wang

Additional information is available at the end of the chapter

http://dx.doi.org/10.5772/59299

1. Introduction

1.1. Classical renin-angiotensin system

The renin–angiotensin system (RAS) is an endocrine system that governs body fluid, electrolyte balance and blood pressure. Within the classical RAS, angiotensinogen (AGT) secreted by liver is enzymatically cleaved to angiotensin (ANG) I by kidney-derived renin. ANG I is, hereafter, cleaved by angiotensin-converting enzyme (ACE) to generate the effector hormone ANG II, which exerts various biological actions through its receptors, ANG II type 1 receptor (AT1) and ANG II type 2 receptor (AT2). The initial reaction between the enzyme renin and the substrate AGT is the rate-limiting step of the RAS [1].

As the RAS is a hormonal cascade that is thought to act as a master controller of blood pressure and fluid balance within the body [2], the systematic RAS has been an important target of antihypertensive medications. There are several groups of drugs in this category that affect different parts of the RAS axis, including ACE inhibitors (ACEI) and angiotensin receptor blockers (ARB), both of which are widely used for anti-hypertension treatment [3]. Additionally, Aliskiren, the first orally active direct renin inhibitor approved for clinical use, is a small molecule competitive inhibitor that specifically inhibits the enzymatic activity of renin [4, 5], consequently it could effectively suppress the rate-limiting step within RAS cascade to reduce the production of ANG II. The recent evidences have shown the effective blood pressure control of Aliskiren, generally well tolerated as monotherapy or in combination with other antihypertensive drugs [3, 6].

2. Tissue renin–angiotensin system

From an evolutionary point of view, it is cost-effective to have a common system to potentiate and effect the actions of the regulating hormones. Interestingly, the RAS is also found in primitive animals without a closed circulatory system, which indicates that the system is far more than a mediator of vasoconstriction [7]. It is now evident that the components of RAS, in addition to the classical pathway, are produced and acting locally in multiple tissues, a concept known as tissue RAS [7]. The local effects of tissue RAS are diverse and depend on the specific tissues involved.

The functional tissue RAS is postulated to participate in various physiological and pathological processes such as insulin secretion [8], glomerular sclerosis [9], renal inflammation [10], atherosclerosis [11], cardiac hypertrophy [12], brain ischemia [13] and follicular development and endometrial cancer in female reproductive tract [14]. A growing body of studies has demonstrated that the diabetic complications, such as cardiovascular disease [15], nephropathy [16] and retinopathy [17], are caused by the high activity of tissue RAS and the increased production of ANG II in local tissues, and the clinical practice has revealed that these pathological alterations associated with diabetes were significantly improved in response to the treatment with RAS inhibitors [15-17]. Additionally, hyperglycemia, obesity, hypertension, and cortisol, well-known risk factors of metabolic disease, are all stimulators on tissue RAS, whereas glucagon-like peptide-1, vitamin D, and aerobic exercise could, to some extent, prevent metabolic disease through inhibiting tissue RAS [7]. Thus, the factors and drugs suppressing tissue RAS activity have potential in improving RAS-involved tissue injuries.

Recent in vivo studies showed that the components of RAS, such as renin, ACE, and ANG II receptors, were expressed in the local milieu of bone [1, 18-20], and in vitro study identified the expression of ANG II receptors in primary osteoblasts derived from newborn mouse calvaria [1], indicating the components of RAS are expressed locally in bone microenvironment. Our further animal studies demonstrated that the local RAS in bone was involved in age-related osteoporosis of aging mice [21], and bone deteriorations of mice with either obstructive nephropathy [22] or type 1 diabetes [23]. Other groups elucidated the involvement of skeletal RAS in the process of fracture healing in a mouse femur fracture model [24], and the steroid-induced osteonecrosis in rabbits [20] as well as the development of postmenopausal osteoporosis in ovariectomized (OVX) animal models [25, 26] and glucocorticoid-induced osteoporosis [19]. Therefore, it concludes that the local RAS exists in bone tissue and plays an important role in local bone metabolism.

3. Action of angiotensin II on bone

ANG II has been postulated to be able to act upon the cells involved in bone metabolism through receptors located in osteoblasts and osteoclasts or regulate blood flow in bone marrow capillaries. At the end of last century, the studies showed that ANG II stimulated DNA and collagen synthesis and decreased alkaline phosphatase (ALP) activity in bone cell populations derived from calvariae of fetal rat [27] and newborn rat [28]. Similar effects of ANG II were observed in osteoblastic ROS17/2.8 cells [29] and human adult bone cells obtained by collagenase digestion from trabecular bone [27]. The clonal cell analysis, autoradiographic studies, and receptor subtype analysis suggested that ANG II might be intimately involved in the proliferation of the osteoblast-rich populations of cells through the AT1 receptor [27, 28], which also plays one of the essential roles in bone metabolism as a mechanoreceptor of osteoblasts [30].

When investigating the direct effects of ANG II on matured osteoblasts, the results revealed that ANG II inhibited the expression of mRNA for osteocalcin, which is a protein that is specifically expressed during maturation of osteoblastic cells, decreased the activity of ALP, the number and the total area of mineralized nodules as well as reduced the accumulation of calcium in cells and the matrix layer [31]. Besides, the ANG II-involved impairment of bone formation may be attributed that it altered the expression of Cbfa1 by activating the cAMP signaling pathway and subsequently reduced osteoblast number and osteoblastic function [32]. SOST, which encodes sclerostin, is a secretory product of osteocytes that counters Wnt signaling, thereby negatively regulates bone formation [33]. The AT1-involved inhibition on bone formation was highly correlated with its regulation on downstream factor SOST, as the decreased SOST expression in osteocytes was observed in AT1-deficient mice [34]. Furthermore, the treatment with ANG II strikingly increased the expressions of matrix metalloproteinase (MMP)-3 and-13 through MAPK signaling pathways via the AT1 in osteoblastic ROS17/2.8 cells, suggesting that ANG II stimulated the degradation process that occurs during extracellular matrix (ECM) turnover in osteoid by increasing the production of MMP-3 and-13 in osteoblasts [29]. Additionally, ANG II induced mitochondrial dysfunction and promoted apoptosis via JNK signaling pathway in primary mouse calvaria osteoblast [35]. Taken together, the target genes including Cbfa1, SOST, MMP-3 and MMP-13, and the signaling pathways like MAPK and JNK are involved in the mediation of ANG II on osteoblastic function and bone formation.

Osteoblast modulates osteoclast differentiation by producing both positive and negative regulators, most notably receptor activator of NF-κB ligand (RANKL) and osteoprotegerin (OPG), respectively [36]. Of note, it has been recently found that ANG II could induce the differentiation of bone marrow mononuclear cells to multinuclear cells and the number of multinuclear cells in osteoclasts as well as increase tartrate-resistant acid phosphatase (TRAP)-positive multinuclear osteoclasts due to its stimulation on the expression of osteoclastogenesis-supporting cytokine, RANKL in osteoblasts, leading to the activation of osteoclasts [1, 25], whereas these effects were completely blocked by either ANG II type 1 receptor blockade (olmesartan) or mitogen-activated protein kinase kinase inhibitors (U0126) [25]. Importantly, ANG II itself had no capacity to induce osteoclast differentiation and did not potentiate osteoclast formation triggered by RANKL, while it stimulated the formation of osteoclasts in the co-culture system of primary osteoblasts and bone marrow macrophages in a dose-dependent manner [1, 32]. Taken together, these results suggested that ANG II stimulates osteoclastogenesis by acting on osteoblastic cells (i.e., 'the soil cells'), but not through a direct action on hematopoietic 'seed cells' [1].

It was found that the TRAP activity and the TRAP-positive stained area were significantly increased in the tibia of OVX rats with systemic administration of ANG II at a subpresser dose (200 ng/kg/min), and the treatment with ANG II significantly induced the ovariectomy-induced increase in urinary level of deoxypyridinoline [25]. The ratio of ALP to TRAP was significantly decreased in the tibia of OVX rats upon to ANG II treatment. These results suggested that ANG II accelerated the turnover of bone metabolism, which is similar to the typical pattern in elderly postmenopausal women who are at high risk for osteoporosis [25]. Of importance, the bone density as assessed by double energy X ray absorptiometry (DEXA) was significantly decreased in the tibia of OVX rats by ANG II. These results suggested that ANG II directly accelerated estrogen deficiency-induced osteoporosis.

4. Interaction of AT1 and AT2 on bone

Previous studies have focused on the ANG II–AT1 interactions since these are the best described and considered the most important. However, the system is complex and several other components probably play significant roles as well [7]. Several publications raise the possibility that AT1 and AT2 carry out negative cross-talk within fibroblasts and vascular endothelial cells with respect to each other's signaling pathways and responses [37]. This may be of particular importance when the AT1 are pharmacologically blocked.

Asaba et al. determined the relative contribution of the two receptors for transducing the osteoclastogenesis-supporting function of ANG II in osteoblasts by knocking down the expression of each of the receptors with siRNA in primary osteoblasts in culture [1]. In AT1-knockdown osteoblasts, the stimulatory effect of ANG II on osteoclast formation was somewhat enhanced. In AT2-knockdown osteoblasts, in contrast, the osteoclastogenic potential was markedly attenuated [1], which was consistent with that AT2 deficiency increased bone mass of distal metaphyseal regions of femoral in mice as well as the treatment with AT2 blocker PD123319 suppressed ANG II-induced increase in the number of osteoclasts in organ cultures of bone [18]. *Asaba* et al.'s study suggested that the action of ANG II on osteoblasts in terms of stimulating osteoclastogenesis was mainly mediated through the AT2 and AT1 might exert an inhibitory effect on AT2. These findings in osteoblasts are consistent with the notion that the functions of AT1 and AT2 are in many cases counter-regulatory to each other [7]. However, they are contrary to the conclusion that AT2 is the protective arm of RAS and counterbalances pathological processes and enable recovery from disease [38]. Thus, further studies are needed to dissect the signaling pathways downstream of each receptor in osteoblasts.

5. ACE inhibitors and osteoporosis

Osteoporosis, hypertension, diabetes are major chronic diseases in older subjects and the latter two are well known to be high risk factors for osteoporosis. As ACE inhibitors are usually prescribed for hypertension, cardiac failure, and diabetic nephropathy [23, 39], it is important to know the prospective effects of ACEI on bones of these patients taking ACEI treatment.

Previously, most of clinical studies demonstrated that patients treated with ACEI showed an increased bone mineral density (BMD) and a reduced fracture risk [40-45]. The menopausal and hypertensive women who followed treatment with ACEI fosinopril did not present the physiological loss of bone mass that affected to menopausal women without treatment [43]. A large case–control analysis carried out in the UK, suggested a possibly decreased fracture risk associated with longer-term use of ACE inhibitors [40], and in an open prospective study including 134 patients with low to moderate hypertension and stable BMD, the plasma calcium and 25-hydroxyvitamin D levels were both increased in patients treated with the ACEI quinapril [41]. It also significantly increased BMD of lumbar spine in female subjects with ACE DD genotype, which could induce a higher level of ANG II [41]. The research group from Hong Kong performed two large scale cohort studies which investigated the risk factors for osteoporotic fractures in Hong Kong-dwelling elderly Chinese, and their data concluded that male ACEI users had higher BMD at the total hip, female neck and lumbar spine than non-users. Likewise, female ACEI users also had higher BMD than non-users, although only significant at the femoral neck [42].

While, in the contrary to the above mentioned beneficial effects of ACEI on bone health, the recent emerging evidences indicated that ACEI use did not change the rate and risk of fracture [46], and even led to greater bone loss [39, 47, 48]. The same research group from Hong Kong recently also stated that female continuous users of ACEI had increased bone loss both in total hip and femur neck [47]. A large sample size study in American men also supported this theory by showing that ACEI use was associated with increased bone loss [39], moreover, another prospective study-a cohort study of atomic bomb survivors in Japan, demonstrated that ACEI use was associated with increased bone loss of femoral neck in older Japanese [48].

Similarly in animal studies, the use of ACEI enalapril (10-20 mg/kg, i.g.) did not show positive effects on bone function of OVX mice [49] or OVX spontaneously hypertensive rats (SHR) [50], and the administration of enalapril (0.4 mg/kg, i.p.) in a dose recommended for the treatment of hypertension did not cause significant changes in bone density, the ash and mineral content or morphometric parameters of the femur in female Wistar rats [51]. Another ACEI moexipril, when given alone at oral dose of 10 mg/kg, had no effect on the cancellous bone site in either OVX or sham-operated rats and did not hamper the osteoprotective effects of 17beta-estradiol [52]. Even though the treatment of Tsukuba hypertensive mouse with enalapril improved osteoporosis [1] as well as the OVX rats in response to the treatment with ACEI captopril (1 or 5 mg/kg) showed the increased trabecular area of lumbar vertebrae (L4) and the improved biomechanical properties by increasing L5 break stress and elastic modulus [26], our recent published article elucidated that the treatment with captopril (10 mg/kg, i.g.) significantly elevated serum level of TRAP 5b, and had a trend to decrease BMD of trabecular bone and damage micro-architecture of proximal tibial head and distal femoral end in type 1 diabetic mice [23].

Based on the facts that ANG II locally in bone tissue has detrimental effects to bone function and ACE is the major enzyme producing ANG II, it is surprising that ACEI could not improve even accelerate bone loss in both humans and animals. Since the modest changes in ACE level affect the levels of its substrates much more than its products, indicating that relatively small changes in the levels of ACE affect kinin level more than ANG II level [53], a possible reason comes from the regulation of ACE on kinin-kallikrein system within which bradykinin can stimulate bone resorption and reduce BMD [47]. Another possible explanation we should consider is that although short-term ACEI therapy was associated with decreased ANG II level, there were some evidences that long-term ACE inhibition resulted in a return of ANG II towards baseline level, so-called 'ACE escape' [47]. The complete mechanisms have not yet been fully demonstrated. More research needs to be carried out to clarify the influence of the ACEI treatment on bone health as this might be of clinical relevance when antihypertensive therapy is initiated, particularly in hypertensive women who typically suffer from a concomitant rapid onset of osteoporosis after menopause [52].

6. Angiotensin receptor blockers and osteoporosis

The clinical profiles of users of ACEI and ARB were very similar. In the USA, ARB was usually prescribed when ACEI was not tolerated, thus explaining the smaller number of ARB users [39] and limited human studies of ARB and BMD or fracture risk in the literatures [46]. The completed studies on the affections of ARB on bone function in human and animals have shown contradictory results.

The recent population-based, retrospective cohort study with propensity score-matching using administrative databases in Ontario, Canada to examine the risk of osteoporosis-related fractures in hypertensive elderly patients treated with ARBs versus ACEIs, showed that there was no significant difference between the effects of ARBs and ACE inhibitors on hip and other osteoporotic fractures [54]. A large cohort study on Medicare beneficiaries with a diagnosis of hypertension initiating single-drug therapy for anti-hypertension treatment suggested the increasingly protective effect of ARB on relative fracture risk over time [46]. While, the study with large sample size of community-dwelling older adults from six different geographic regions demonstrated that the use of ARBs did not have any significant overall effect on bone loss in older men [39].

The contradictory results about the actions of ARBs on bone metabolism were also shown among animal studies. The treatment with telmisartan, olmesartan, and losartan, could reduce bone loss of OVX mice [49], attenuate the ovariectomy-induced decrease in BMD [25], and increase bone strength, mass and trabecular connections of OVX rats femur [55, 56], respectively. Moreover, telmisartan partially protected from thiazolidinedione-induced bone loss by actively blocking thiazolidinedione-induced anti-osteoblastic activity via maintaining PPARγ serine 112 phosphorylation [57], and promoted fracture healing in a mice model [58]. However, some studies reported ARBs did not cause significant changes of bone properties in normal female rats [51], type 2 diabetic mice [57], OVX rats [59] or orchiectomized rats [60]. Importantly, it was noted that in some animal models ARBs may lead to more bone injuries [1, 61]. The treatment of transgenic Tsukuba hypertensive mouse with losartan resulted in exacerbation of the low bone mass phenotype [1]. The study in our group demonstrated a trend of losartan to promote the loss of bone mass and the deteriorations of trabecular bone micro-architecture in type 1 diabetic mice due to the compensatory stimulation of bone RAS activation as shown by the up-regulation of renin and ANG II expression in bone tissue [61].

7. Perspective

It has been argued that neither ACEIs nor ARBs completely block the RAS cascade due to the disruption of the feedback inhibition of renin production [62]. The increase in renin activity stimulates the conversion of ANG I and ultimately ANG II, which largely limits the efficacy of RAS inhibition [63]. The increased renin can also act through the prorenin/renin receptor, which may cause tissue damages independent of ANG II [64]. Thus, as compared to single treatment with RAS inhibitors, whether combining renin inhibitor, like Aliskiren, with ARB or ACEI could generate better therapeutic effects on tissue injuries, such as osteoporosis, should be further clarified.

As discussed in this chapter, RAS locally plays a key role in the modulation of bone metabolism. However, over the past 10 years, several studies have presented evidences for the existence of a new arm of the RAS, namely the ACE2/ANG-(1–7)/Mas axis [65]. The identification of the ACE homolog, ACE2 as a key ANG-(1–7)-forming enzyme, unravels the existence of a distinct enzymatic pathway for the production of ANG-(1-7), which has a broad range of effects in different organs and tissues that goes beyond its initially described cardiovascular and renal actions [66]. This heptapeptide exerts its actions through binding to a G protein-coupled receptor Mas, distinct from AT1 and AT2 [67]. It is now accepted that the ACE2/ANG-(1–7)/Mas axis is able to counteract most of the deleterious actions of the ACE/ANG II/AT1 axis, especially in pathological conditions [68] such as cardiac dysfunction, increased blood pressure, decreased baroreflex function, endothelial dysfunction, reduced reproductive function, increased thrombogenesis [66]. Thus, how the cross-talk and the interaction between the dual axis systems of RAS contribute to the maintainance of bone metabolism needs to be further investigated and elucidated for better understanding the molecular mechanism of bone metabolic diseases.

Acknowledgements

This work was sponsored by National Natural Science Foundation of China (No. 81202894).

Author details

Yan Zhang[1*] and Liang Wang[2]

*Address all correspondence to: medicineyan@aliyun.com

1 Center for Systems Biomedical Sciences, University of Shanghai for Science and Technology, Shanghai, China

2 Department of Orthopaedics, The 309th hospital of Chinese People's Liberation Army, Beijing, China

References

[1] Asaba Y, Ito M, Fumoto T, Watanabe K, Fukuhara R, Takeshita S, Nimura Y, Ishida J, Fukamizu A, Ikeda K. Activation of renin-angiotensin system induces osteoporosis independently of hypertension. J Bone Miner Res 2009;24(2) 241-250.

[2] Namazi S, Ardeshir-Rouhani-Fard S, Abedtash H. The effect of renin angiotensin system on tamoxifen resistance. Med Hypotheses 2011;77(1) 152-155.

[3] Robles NR, Cerezo I, Hernandez-Gallego R. Renin-angiotensin system blocking drugs. J Cardiovasc Pharmacol Ther 2014;19(1) 14-33.

[4] Wood JM, Maibaum J, Rahuel J, Grütter MG, Cohen NC, Rasetti V, Rüger H, Göschke R, Stutz S, Fuhrer W, Schilling W, Rigollier P, Yamaguchi Y, Cumin F, Baum HP, Schnell CR, Herold P, Mah R, Jensen C, O'Brien E, Stanton A, Bedigian MP. Structure-based design of aliskiren, a novel orally effective renin inhibitor. Biochem Biophys Res Commun 2003;308(4) 698-705.

[5] Zhang Y, Wang Y, Chen Y, Deb DK, Sun T, Zhao Q, Li YC. Inhibition of renin activity by aliskiren ameliorates diabetic nephropathy in type 1 diabetes mouse model. J Diabetes Mellitus 2012;2(3) 353-360.

[6] Sen S, Sabırlı S, Ozyiğit T, Uresin Y. Aliskiren: review of efficacy and safety data with focus on past and recent clinical trials. Ther Adv Chronic Dis 2013;4(5) 232-241.

[7] Skov J, Persson F, Frøkiær J, Christiansen JS. Tissue renin-angiotensin systems: a unifying hypothesis of metabolic disease. Front Endocrinol (Lausanne) 2014;5 23.

[8] Lau T, Carlsson PO, Leung PS. Evidence for a local angiotensin-generating system and dose-dependent inhibition of glucose-stimulated insulin release by angiotensin II in isolated pancreatic islets. Diabetologia 2004;47(2) 240-248.

[9] Zhang Z, Zhang Y, Ning G, Deb DK, Kong J, Li YC. Combination therapy with AT1 receptor blocker and vitamin D analog markedly ameliorates diabetic nephropathy. Proc Natl Acad Sci USA 2008;105(41) 15896-15901.

[10] Zhang Y, Deb DK, Kong J, Ning G, Wang Y, Li G, Chen Y, Zhang Z, Strugnell S, Sabbagh Y, Arbeeny C, Li YC. Long-term therapeutic effect of vitamin D analog Doxercalciferol on diabetic nephropathy: strong synergism with AT1 receptor antagonist. Am J Physiol Renal Physiol 2009;297(3) F791-F801.

[11] Koïtka A, Cao Z, Koh P, Watson AMD, Sourris KC, Loufrani L, Soro-Paavonen A, Walther T, Woollard KJ, Jandeleit-Dahm KA, Cooper ME, Allen TJ. Angiotensin II subtype 2 receptor blockade and deficiency attenuate the development of atherosclerosis in an apolipoprotein E-deficient mouse model of diabetes. Diabetologia 2010;53(3) 584-592.

[12] Inaba S, Iwai M, Furuno M, Kanno H, Senba I, Okayama H, Mogi M, Higaki J, Horiuchi M. Role of angiotensin-converting enzyme 2 in cardiac hypertrophy induced by nitric oxide synthase inhibition. J Hypertens 2011;29(11) 2236-2245.

[13] Jiang T, Gao L, Lu J, Zhang YD. ACE2-Ang-(1-7)-Mas axis in brain: A potential target for prevention and treatment of ischemic stroke. Curr Neuropharmacol 2013;11(2) 209-217.

[14] Herr D, Bekes I, Wulff C. Local renin-angiotensin system in the reproductive system. Front Endocrinol (Lausanne) 2013;4 150.

[15] Vijan SG. Angiotensin-converting enzyme inhibitors (ACEIs), not angiotensin receptor blockers (ARBs), are preferred and effective mode of therapy in high cardiovascular risk patients. J Indian Med Assoc 2009;107(3) 178-182.

[16] Hoogwerf BJ. Renin-angiotensin system blockade and cardiovascular and renal protection. Am J Cardiol 2010;105(1 Suppl) 30A-35A.

[17] Wright AD, Dodson PM. Diabetic retinopathy and blockade of the renin-angiotensin system: new data from the DIRECT study programme. Eye (Lond) 2007;24(1) 1-6.

[18] Izu Y, Mizoguchi F, Kawamata A, Hayata T, Nakamoto T, Nakashima K, Inagami T, Ezura Y, Noda M. Angiotensin II type 2 receptor blockade increases bone mass. J Biol Chem 2009;284(8) 4857-4864.

[19] Yongtao Z, Kunzheng W, Jingjing Z, Hu S, Jianqiang K, Ruiyu L, Chunsheng W. Glucocorticoids activate the local renin-angiotensin system in bone: possible mechanism for glucocorticoid-induced osteoporosis. Endocrine 2014;DOI: 10.1007/s12020-014-0196-z.

[20] Zhang Y, Wang K, Song Q, Liu R, Ji W, Ji L, Wang C. Role of the local bone renin-angiotensin system in steroid-induced osteonecrosis in rabbits. Mol Med Rep 2014;9(4) 1128-1134.

[21] Gu SS, Zhang Y, Li XL, Wu SY, Diao TY, Hai R, Deng H. Involvement of the skeletal renin-angiotensin system in age-related osteoporosis of ageing mice. Biosci Biotechnol Biochem 2012;76(7) 1367-1371.

[22] Gu SS, Zhang Y, Wu SY, Diao TY, Gebru YA, Deng H. Early molecular responses of bone to obstructive nephropathy induced by unilateral ureteral obstruction in mice. Nephrology 2012;17(8) 767-773.

[23] Diao TY, Pan H, Gu SS, Chen X, Zhang FY, Wong MS, Zhang Y. Effects of angiotensin-converting enzyme inhibitor, captopril, on bone of mice with streptozotocin-induced type 1 diabetes. J Bone Miner Metab 2014;32(3) 261-270.

[24] Garcia P, Schwenzer S, Slotta JE, Scheuer C, Tami AE, Holstein JH, Histing T, Burkhardt M, Pohlemann T, Menger MD. Inhibition of angiotensin-converting enzyme stimulates fracture healing and periosteal callus formation-role of a local renin-angiotensin system. Br J Pharmacol 2010; 159(8) 1672-1680.

[25] Shimizu H, Nakagami H, Osako MK, Hanayama R, Kunugiza Y, Kizawa T, Tomita T, Yoshikawa H, Ogihara T, Morishita R. Angiotensin II accelerates osteoporosis by activating osteoclasts. FASEB J 2008;22(7) 2465-2475.

[26] Liu YY, Yao WM, Wu T, Xu BL, Chen F, Cui L. Captopril improves osteopenia in ovariectomized rats and promotes bone formation in osteoblasts. J Bone Miner Metab 2011;29(2) 149-158.

[27] Lamparter S, Kling L, Schrader M, Ziegler R, Pfeilschifter J. Effects of angiotensin II on bone cells in vitro. J Cell Physiol 1998;175(1) 89-98.

[28] Hiruma Y, Inoue A, Hirose S, Hagiwara H. Angiotensin II stimulates the proliferation of osteoblast-rich populations of cells from rat calvariae. Biochem Biophys Res Commun 1997;230(1) 176-178.

[29] Nakai K, Kawato T, Morita T, Iinuma T, Kamio N, Zhao N, Maeno M. Angiotensin II induces the production of MMP-3 and MMP-13 through the MAPK signaling pathways via the AT(1) receptor in osteoblasts. Biochimie 2013;95(4) 922-933.

[30] Bandow K, Nishikawa Y, Ohnishi T, Kakimoto K, Soejima K, Iwabuchi S, Kuroe K, Matsuguchi T. Low-intensity pulsed ultrasound (LIPUS) induces RANKL, MCP-1, and MIP-1beta expression in osteoblasts through the angiotensin II type 1 receptor. J Cell Physiol 2007;211(2) 392-398.

[31] Hagiwara H, Hiruma Y, Inoue A, Yamaguchi A, Hirose S. Deceleration by angiotensin II of the differentiation and bone formation of rat calvarial osteoblastic cells. J Endocrinol 1998;156(3) 543-550.

[32] Guan XX, Zhou Y, Li JY. Reciprocal roles of angiotensin II and Angiotensin II Receptors Blockade (ARB) in regulating Cbfa1/RANKL via cAMP signaling pathway: possible mechanism for hypertension-related osteoporosis and antagonistic effect of ARB on hypertension-related osteoporosis. Int J Mol Sci 2011;12(7) 4206-4213.

[33] Paszty C, Turner CH, Robinson MK. Sclerostin: a gem from the genome leads to bone-building antibodies. J Bone Miner Res 2010;25(9) 1897-1904.

[34] Kaneko K, Ito M, Fumoto T, Fukuhara R, Ishida J, Fukamizu A, Ikeda K. Physiological function of the angiotensin AT1a receptor in bone remodeling. J Bone Miner Res 2011;26(12) 2959-2966.

[35] Li G, Wang M, Hao L, Loo WT, Jin L, Cheung MN, Chow LW, Ng EL. Angiotensin II induces mitochondrial dysfunction and promotes apoptosis via JNK signalling pathway in primary mouse calvaria osteoblast. Arch Oral Biol 2014;59(5) 513-523.

[36] Zhang Y, Dong XL, Leung PC, Wong MS. Differential mRNA expression profiles in proximal tibia of aged rats in response to ovariectomy and low-Ca diet. Bone 2009;44(1) 46-52.

[37] Yayama K, Okamoto H. Angiotensin II-induced vasodilation via type 2 receptor: role of bradykinin and nitric oxide. Int Immunopharmacol 2008;8(2) 312-318.

[38] Namsolleck P, Recarti C, Foulquier S, Steckelings UM, Unger T. AT(2) receptor and tissue injury: therapeutic implications. Curr Hypertens Rep 2014;16(2) 416.

[39] Kwok T, Leung J, Zhang YF, Bauer D, Ensrud KE, Barrett-Connor E, Leung PC; Osteoporotic Fractures inMen(MrOS) Research Group. Does the use of ACE inhibitors or angiotensin receptor blockers affect bone loss in older men? Osteoporos Int 2012;23(8) 2159-2167.

[40] Schlienger RG, Kraenzlin ME, Jick SS, Meier CR. Use of beta-blockers and risk of fractures. JAMA 2004;292(11) 1326-1332.

[41] Pérez-Castrillón JL, Silva J, Justo I, Sanz A, Martín-Luquero M, Igea R, Escudero P, Pueyo C, Díaz C, Hernández G, Dueñas A. Effect of quinapril, quinapril-hydrochlorothiazide, and enalapril on the bone mass of hypertensive subjects: relationship with angiotensin converting enzyme polymorphisms. Am J Hypertens 2003;16(6) 453-459.

[42] Lynn H, Kwok T, Wong SY, Woo J, Leung PC. Angiotensin converting enzyme inhibitor use is associated with higher bone mineral density in elderly Chinese. Bone 2006;38(4) 584-588.

[43] García-Testal A, Monzó A, Rabanaque G, González A, Romeu A. Evolution of the bone mass of hypertense menopausal women in treatment with fosinopril. Med Clin (Barc) 2006;127(18) 692-694.

[44] Rejnmark L, Vestergaard P, Mosekilde L. Treatment with beta-blockers, ACE inhibitors, and calcium-channel blockers is associated with a reduced fracture risk: a nationwide case-control study. J Hypertens 2006;24(3) 581-589.

[45] Ghosh M, Majumdar SR. Antihypertensive medications, bone mineral density, and fractures: a review of old cardiac drugs that provides new insights into osteoporosis. Endocrine 2014;46(3) 397-405.

[46] Solomon DH, Mogun H, Garneau K, Fischer MA. Risk of fractures in older adults using antihypertensive medications. J Bone Miner Res 2011;26(7) 1561-1567.

[47] Zhang YF, Qin L, Leung PC, Kwok TC. The effect of angiotensin-converting enzyme inhibitor use on bone loss in elderly Chinese. J Bone Miner Metab 2012;30(6) 666-673.

[48] Masunari N, Fujiwara S, Nakata Y, Furukawa K, Kasagi F. Effect of angiotensin converting enzyme inhibitor and benzodiazepine intake on bone loss in older Japanese. Hiroshima J Med Sci 2008;57(1) 17-25.

[49] Kang KY, Kang Y, Kim M, Kim Y, Yi H, Kim J, Jung HR, Park SH, Kim HY, Ju JH, Hong YS. The effects of antihypertensive drugs on bone mineral density in ovariectomized mice. J Korean Med Sci 2013;28(8) 1139-1144.

[50] Ma YF, Stimpel M, Liang H, Pun S, Jee WS. Impact of antihypertensive therapy on the skeleton: effects of moexipril and hydrochlorothiazide on osteopenia in spontaneously hypertensive ovariectomized rats. J Endocrinol 1997;154(3) 467-474.

[51] Broulík PD, Tesar V, Zima T, Jirsa M. Impact of antihypertensive therapy on the skeleton: effects of enalapril and AT1 receptor antagonist losartan in female rats. Physiol Res 2001;50(4) 353-358.

[52] Stimpel M, Jee WS, Ma Y, Yamamoto N, Chen Y. Impact of antihypertensive therapy on postmenopausal osteoporosis: effects of the angiotensin converting enzyme inhibitor moexipril, 17beta-estradiol and their combination on the ovariectomy-induced cancellous bone loss in young rats. J Hypertens 1995;13(12 Pt 2) 1852-1856.

[53] Kakoki M, Sullivan KA, Backus C, Hayes JM, Oh SS, Hua K, Gasim AM, Tomita H, Grant R, Nossov SB, Kim HS, Jennette JC, Feldman EL, Smithies O. Lack of both bradykinin B1 and B2 receptors enhances nephropathy, neuropathy, and bone mineral loss in Akita diabetic mice. Proc Natl Acad Sci U S A 2010;107(22) 10190-10195.

[54] Butt DA, Mamdani M, Gomes T, Lix L, Lu H, Tu K; On Behalf of the Hypertension Outcome, Surveillance Team. Risk of osteoporotic fractures with angiotensin II receptor blockers versus angiotensin converting-enzyme inhibitors in hypertensive community-dwelling elderly. J Bone Miner Res 2014;DOI: 10.1002/jbmr.2271.

[55] Donmez BO, Ozdemir S, Sarikanat M, Yaras N, Koc P, Demir N, Karayalcin B, Oguz N. Effect of angiotensin II type 1 receptor blocker on osteoporotic rat femurs. Pharmacol Rep 2012;64(4) 878-888.

[56] Rajkumar DS, Faitelson AV, Gudyrev OS, Dubrovin GM, Pokrovski MV, Ivanov AV. Comparative evaluation of enalapril and losartan in pharmacological correction of experimental osteoporosis and fractures of its background. J Osteoporos 2013;2013 325693.

[57] Kolli V, Stechschulte LA, Dowling AR, Rahman S, Czernik PJ, Lecka-Czernik B. Partial agonist, telmisartan, maintains PPARγ serine 112 phosphorylation, and does not affect osteoblast differentiation and bone mass. PLoS One 2014;9(5) e96323.

[58] Zhao X, Wang JX, Feng YF, Wu ZX, Zhang Y, Shi L, Tan QC, Yan YB, Lei W. Systemic treatment with telmisartan improves femur fracture healing in mice. PLoS One 2014;9(3) e92085.

[59] Li YQ, Ji H, Shen Y, Ding LJ, Zhuang P, Yang YL, Huang QJ. Chronic treatment with angiotensin AT1 receptor antagonists reduced serum but not bone TGF-beta1 levels in ovariectomized rats. Can J Physiol Pharmacol 2009;87(1) 51-55.

[60] Zhang YF, Qin L, Kwok TC, Yeung BH, Li GD, Liu F. Effect of angiotensin II type I receptor blocker losartan on bone deterioration in orchiectomized male hypertensive and normotensive rats. Chin Med J (Engl) 2013;126(14) 2661-2665.

[61] Zhang Y, Diao TY, Gu SS, Wu SY, Gebru YA, Chen X, Wang JY, Ran S, Wong MS. Effects of angiotensin II type 1 receptor blocker on bones in mice with type 1 diabetes induced by streptozotocin. J Renin Angiotensin Aldosterone Syst 2014;15(3) 218-227.

[62] Koid SS, Ziogas J, Campbell DJ. Aliskiren reduces myocardial ischemia-reperfusion injury by a bradykinin B2 receptor-and angiotensin AT2 receptor-mediated mechanism. Hypertension 2014;63(4) 768-773.

[63] Zhang Z, Zhang Y, Ning G, Kong J, Deb DK, Li YC. Combination therapy with AT1 receptor blocker and vitamin D analog markedly ameliorates diabetic nephropathy. Proc Natl Acad Sci U S A 2008;105(41) 15896-15901.

[64] Zhang Y, Deb DK, Kong J, Ning G, Wang Y, Li G, Chen Y, Zhang Z, Strugnell S, Sabbagh Y, Arbeeny C, Li YC. Long-term therapeutic effect of vitamin D analog Doxercalciferol on diabetic nephropathy: strong synergism with AT1 receptor antagonist. Am J Physiol Renal Physiol 2009;297(3) F791-F801.

[65] Passos-Silva DG, Verano-Braga T, Santos RA. Angiotensin-(1-7): beyond the cardiorenal actions. Clin Sci (Lond) 2013;124(7) 443-456.

[66] Santos RA, Ferreira AJ, Verano-Braga T, Bader M. Angiotensin-converting enzyme 2, angiotensin-(1-7) and Mas: new players of the renin-angiotensin system. J Endocrinol 2013;216(2) R1-R17.

[67] Horiuchi M, Iwanami J, Mogi M. Regulation of angiotensin II receptors beyond the classical pathway. Clin Sci (Lond) 2012;123(4) 193-203.

[68] Wong TP, Ho KY, Ng EK, Debnam ES, Leung PS. Upregulation of ACE2-ANG-(1-7)-Mas axis in jejunal enterocytes of type 1 diabetic rats: implications for glucose transport. Am J Physiol Endocrinol Metab 2012;303(5) E669-E681.

Chapter 6

Pharmacological Treatment of Osteoporosis

Jorge Malouf, Berta Magallares and Roberto Güerri

Additional information is available at the end of the chapter

http://dx.doi.org/10.5772/59469

1. Introduction

Osteoporosis can be divided into two principle strands, clinical osteoporosis and densitometric osteoporosis. Clinical osteoporosis involves the identification of a fragility fracture and does not need densitometry for treatment to begin. Densitometric osteoporosis is identified via an assessment of bone mineral density. Approaches to treatment depend on the global fracture risk and the outcomes of densitometric tests.

The initial stage of the pharmacological treatment of osteoporosis is to identify the pathology of the primary condition or to determine whether the loss of bone density is a secondary symptom of a separate condition. Where secondary osteoporosis is identified, priority is given to the treatment of the primary condition. The option of pharmacological therapy must only be contemplated if the risk of fracture is too elevated, given that the intention behind pharmacological treatment in osteoporosis is to reduce the fracture risk. Based on World Health Organization figures, less than half of patients presenting a fragility fracture have been diagnosed with densitometric osteoporosis [1]. Once a course of medication has begun, long-term management must address improvements to lifestyle and take aspects of, security, cost, and compliance into account. As such, it is absolutely necessary to assess and make determinations on the basis of cost, assessment of cost-efficiency, and the adaptability of patients to drug security.

2. Antiresorptives

2.1. Calcitonin

Calcitonin binds to osteoclasts and hinders bone resorption. The use of salmon calcitonin has previously been widespread as a result of its extreme potency in humans, a result of its greater affinity for the human calcitonin receptor.

Calcitonin is now no longer a treatment for osteoporosis, having been supplanted by other treatments. Following a European risk-benefit analysis, the scientific committee of the European Medicines Agency (CHMP) advised that treatments using calcitonin should only be deployed in short-term scenarios.. Treatments using injectable calcitonin should be confined to the short-term in Paget's disease, the prevention of acute bone loss as a result of sudden immobilization and hypercalcemia resulting from cancer. In addition to this, calcitonin has been proven to be effective in treating pain resulting from fractures of the vertebral column. [2-4]

2.2. Hormonal Replacement Therapy (HRT)

HRT is a form of treatment which deploys varying doses of estrogen, sometimes on its own, sometimes in combination with progestagens. The calculated risk of fracture, based on principal cohort trials of postmenopausal women treated with HRT over the long term, indicate an appreciable lowering of the likelihood of both vertebral fracture (RR=0.6; CI 95%: 0.36 to 0.99) and wrist fracture (RR=0.39; CI 95%: 0.24 to 0.64), but a non-significant lowering of the likelihood of hip fracture (RR=0.64; CI 95%: 0.32 to 1.04). The WHI trial (Women's Health Initiative), a randomised clinical trial (RCT) that assessed postmenopausal women randomly assigned to combined HRT (combined equine estrogen 0.625mg daily plus medroxyprogesterone 2.5mg daily) or a placebo, recorded, following 5.2 years of treatment, a decrease in hip fracture risk of 34% (hazard ratio [HR]=0.66; CI 95%: 0.45 to 0.98), in clinical vertebral fractures of 34% (HR=0.66; CI 95%: 0.44 to 0.98) and in any fracture of 24% (HR=0.76; CI 95%: 0.69 to 0.85) [5,6]. In the same investigation, the cohort taking estrogen on its own demonstrated comparable outcomes, however the treatment was put on hold as a result of an adverse risk-benefit ratio. In two meta-analyses of RCT's, a decrease of 27% (RR=0.73; CI 95%: 0.56 to 0.94) in non-vertebral fractures and a trend towards a reduction of vertebral fractures (RR=0.66; CI 95%: 0.41 to 1.07) was recorded [7]. Nonetheless, neither the HERS (The Heart and Estrogen + Progestin Replacement Study) RCT nor the subsequent group, the HERS II study (Hulley et al., 1998), were able to register a decrease of the risk of hip fractures or of other locations (RR=1.04; CI 95%: 0.87 to 1.25) in patients with a history of cardiovascular disease [8].

The British National Institute of Health and Clinical Excellence published a meta-analysis of RCTs on HRT efficacy (with estrogen alone or combined) compared with placebo/non-treatment in postmenopausal women or those with surgical menopause [9]. The outcomes were organised according to the location of the fracture and the RCT used as the basis for the calculation of the relative risk was also identified. The outcomes are outlined in table 1.

Fracture Location	Nr of RCTs	n	RESULTS	References
Vertebral fracture	4 RCTs	11,842	RR=0.55; CI 95%: 0.46 to 0.66	[10-13]
Non-vertebral fracture	3 RCTs	11,774	RR=0.73; CI 95%: 0.65 to 0.81	[10, 11,14]
Hip fracture	2 RCTs	11,745	RR=0.63; CI 95%: 0.42 to 0.93	[11,14]
Any type of fracture	3 RCTs	11,556	RR=0.70; CI 95%: 0.63 to 0.78	[14-16]

Table 1. Relative fracture risk in NICE meta-analysis

2.2.1. Security

2.2.1.1. Vascular illness

A thorough and methodical review of five RCTs looking at HRT with estrogen and two looking at combined HRT estrogen plus progesterone, failed to display compelling variance in the occurrence of acute coronary events (including acute myocardial infarction) between the cohort subject to intervention and the control cohort [7]. A combination of the outcomes of three studies contrasting estrogenic therapy to a placebo [11, 17] reported an odds ratio (OR) of 1.34 (IC 95%: 1.07 to 1.68) for cerebral vascular events. The combined outcomes of the studies that contrasted estrogen plus progesterone combined treatment with a placebo [5, 18], indicated an elevated risk of ictus (OR=1.28; CI 95%: 1.05 to 1.57) in the cohort subject to intervention. Out of four thorough and methodical reviews of observational trials looking at women treated with HRT [19-22], three of these indicated a significant decrease in the global mortality risk for acute coronary events. A recently published, thorough and methodical review, that compensated for selection bias of inclusion and analysis, did not reveal any link between the THS and the incidence, and mortality of acute coronary events [22].

The WHI primary prevention trial indicated a distinct elevation of the risk of acute coronary events (41%), starting the second year of treatment (29 instances in the treatment cohort, compared with 21 instances for 10,000 women per year in the general population) [5]. This elevated risk was greater in non-mortal coronary incidents (RR=1.50; CI 95%: 1.08 to 2.08) than in the mortal coronary incidents (RR=1.20; CI 95%: 0.58 to 2.50). The RCTs of HRT with estrogens alone, in both primary and secondary prevention, failed to indicate any positive impact on cerebrovascular illness [23]. In addition, the WHI study cohort with estrogen indicated an elevated risk of cerebrovascular incidents.

2.2.1.2. Venous thrombotic events

In a thorough and methodical review, McLean et al. indicated that estrogen patients treated with estrogen demonstrate an elevated risk of major venous thromboembolic incidents (OR=1.36; CI 95%: 1.01 to 1.86) compared to the placebo cohort [7]. A further thorough and methodical review assessing the impact of HRT (estrogen with or without progestagens) encompassed 12 studies (3 RCTs, 8 case-control studies and 1 cohort study) and indicated an elevated risk of thromboembolism (RR=2.14; CI 95%: 1.64 to 2.81). This risk was elevated in the first two years of the therapy and it varied according to the dose [24].

2.2.1.3. Breast cancer

A thorough and methodical review of 4 RCTs proved that patients treated with estrogens alone have a lower risk of breast cancer (OR=0.79; CI 95%: 0.66 to 0.93) than those treated with the placebo [7]. On the other hand, patients treated with estrogen and progestin have a higher risk of breast cancer (OR=1.28; CI 95%: 1.03 to 1.60) than those treated with the placebo [5, 18, 24].

Nonetheless the combined HRT cohort of the WHI study presented an elevated risk of invasive breast cancer [5]. This elevated risk occurred following the fourth year of treatment (RR=1.26;

CI 95 %: 1.0 to 1.59), with a propensity to rise in line with the treatment's longevity (38 instances compared with 30 for 10,000 women per year).

2.2.1.4. *Endometrial cancer*

The treatment of estrogen alone elevates the risk of subsequent endometrial hyperplasia and cancer [25,26]. A meta-analysis including 29 observational studies reported a demonstrable elevation of the risk of endometrial cancer, with or without combined estrogens (RR=2.3; CI 95%: 2.1 to 2.5) [20]. This risk is directly related to the treatment's longevity and continues to be raised for a maximum of 5 years or more following the termination of treatment.

2.2.1.5. *Ovarian cancer*

Recently published thorough and methodical reviews of observational trials indicate an elevated incidence of ovarian cancer amongst women undergoing treatment, particularly long-term therapies (more than 10 years) [28,28]. Two cohort trials of postmenopausal women who underwent treatment for a period of more than 10 years corroborate this elevated risk of ovarian cancer (RR=2.2; CI 95%: 1.53 to 3.17), as well as an elevated mortality risk (RR=1.59; CI 95%: 1.13 to 2.25) [29, 30].

We can conclude that HRT is an effective therapy both for postmenopausal osteoporosis and for the management of fracture risk. Nevertheless, even taking this conclusion into account, the use of combined HRT is not recommeneded for periods greater than 5 years, given the possible risk factors linked with treatments using a daily dose equivalent to 50 pg of estradiol. When HRT treatment is indicated, it should be prescribed at a low dosage (equivalent to estrogen transdermal patches of 25 mcg), only using higher doses if it is absolutely essential to do so. Estrogens and progestagens are only advised for the treatment of women with intact uteri. The level of the progestagen dose should be determined on the basis of the estrogen dose. In instances where a hysterectomy was carried out as a result of endometrial cancer, HRT should not involve combined estrogen and progestagens. Continuous combined HRT treatment should only commence following one whole year of menopause.

2.3. Selective Estrogen Receptor Modulators (SERMs)

Selective estrogen receptor modulators are medications with a selective impact on the estrogen receptor. They can function as estrogen receptor (ER) agonists in some tissues while in other tissues functioning as estrogen receptor antagonists. As a result of their selective estrogen-agonist behaviour within a variety of tissues, SERMs may be indicated as an alternative option for the prevention or treatment of conditions like osteoporosis, which are the result of a deficiency of estrogen, where avoiding the negatives effects of estrogens is a priority.

2.3.1. *Differences between SERMs*

At present there are two forms of SERM, which are distinguished by their chemical structure: triphenylethylene derivatives, for example tamoxifen and toremifene, and benzothiophene derivatives, for example raloxifene and bazedoxifene. Tamoxifen and toremifene on the one hand are indicated for use in the treatment of breast cancer. Raloxifene on the other hand is used for the prevention and treatment of osteoporosis and in addition the prevention of breast cancer. All SERMs have been linked with an elevated occurrence of pulmonary thromboembolism and with the start of hot flushes, however they also impact in a positive manner on the lipid profile.

The SERMs vary distinctively with regards to tissue specificity. Bazedoxifene appears to have a lower impact on the uterus than estradiol jointly with raloxifene in animal experiments as a result of reduced estrogen receptor alpha agonistic effects.

2.3.2. Raloxifene

Raloxifene acts as estrogen agonist in bone and other systems but not in reproductive tissue. Many trials have proved the effectiveness of raloxifene for preserving bone in the early postmenopausal phase. In a meta-analysis of seven studies (four treatment and three prevention studies) which looked at the impact of raloxifene versus a placebo on bone mineral density, raloxifene augmented bone mineral density within the lumbar spine following a two year period of treatment [31]. A trial of 601 women, five years following the menopause, who were given a daily dose of 30, 60 or 150mg of raloxifene over two years, indicated an augmentation of their bone mineral density in spine and hip, whereas those subjected to the placebo presented reduced bone mineral density in the same locations [32]. In contrast with the results from the placebo, the average alteration in BMD with 60mg of raloxifene was 2.4% in the spine and 2.4% at the total hip ($p<0.001$ versus placebo). Postmenopausal women presenting low bone mass and osteoporosis were monitored over eight years in the study entitled 'Multiple Outcomes of Raloxifene Evaluation' (MORE, n=7,705) and its sister trial entitled 'Continuing Outcomes Relevant to Evista' (CORE, n=4,011) [33]. In relation to fractures, whilst raloxifene treatment led to a decreased risk of vertebral fracture, it failed to demonstrate a reduced risk of non-vertebral fractures. Nevertheless, in a meta-analysis of RCTs contrasting the effects of raloxifene with those of a placebo, raloxifene typically led to a decreased risk of vertebral fractures in postmenopausal women (OR=0.6; CI 95%: 0.5-0.7).

The results of the MORE trial indicated that, following a raloxifene treatment period of four years, at 60mg per day, the cumulative relative risk of one or more vertebral fractures was 0.64 (IC 95%: 0.53 - 0.76), compared with treatment using a placebo.

Verus placebo, treatment with 60mg of raloxifene was also linked to a decrease of 65% to 78% in occurrences of invasive breast cancer and invasive breast cancer with positive estrogen receptor (both $p <0.05$).

2.3.2.1. Adverse Effects

The MORE and CORE studies reported a link between raloxifene and an elevated incidence (1.7 times) of thromboembolism (TE), versus treatment using a placebo (95% CI: 0.93-3.14; risk difference total of 0.9/1,000 women-years) [34]. In a meta-analysis of nine trials, raloxifene treatment was linked with an elevated incidence of deep venous thrombosis and pulmonary embolism (OR=1.5; CI 95%: 1.1-2.1 and OR=1.9; 95% CI: 1.0-3.5, respectively) [35]. The RUTH trial ('Raloxifene Use for The Heart'), which studied 10,101 postmenopausal women with an average age of 68 and presenting with coronary heart disease, indicated a link between raloxifene and an elevated incidence of fatal stroke (HR=1.49; 95% CI: 1.00-2.24, a rise in the absolute risk of 0.7/1,000 women-years) as well as an elevated risk of thromboembolism (HR=1.44; 95% CI: 1.06-1.95, a rise in the absolute risk of 1.2/1,000 women-years) in comparison with the placebo results. No elevated risk of myocardial infarction or other coronary events was indicated in the RUTH trial. Nevertheless, in line with the observations regarding thromboembolism and pulmonary embolism, the outcomes of a recent review of a sub-cohort of the trial indicated that age had an impact on the occurrence of coronary events. For women of 60 years or under, the rate of occurrence of coronary events was distinctly reduced with raloxifene (50 cases), compared with the placebo group (84 cases; HR=0.59; 95% CI: 0.41 to 0.83, p=0.003). Raloxifene was also linked with an elevated occurrence of hot flushes, especially amongst women with recent menopause onset [36].

We can conclude that raloxifene provides an alternative option within osteoporosis therapies for specific patients. The drug's profile relating to heart disease and breast cancer is sound but its links to an elevated risk of venous thrombosis should be taken into account in its use as a treatment.

2.3.2.2. *Bazedoxifene*

Bazedoxifene is a third-generation SERM. Some key differences have been demonstrated between the generations regarding their impact on the uterus and on breast tissue in particular [37]. The drug was developed with raloxifene as a template and by replacing the benzothiophene core with an indole ring [38].

In a phase II trial of healthy postmenopausal women, oral doses of bazedoxifene 2.5, 5, 10, 20, 30, or 40mg per day were as a rule well-tolerated and did not aggravate the endometrium. In addition, bazedoxifene 30 and 40 mg resulted in a notably reduced increase in the thickness of the endometrium and distinctly lowered the occurrence of uterine bleeding versus results from the placebo. In a two-year phase III trial of postmenopausal women at risk of osteoporosis, bazedoxifene 10, 20, and 40mg were proven to prevent bone loss and decrease bone turnover and were linked with a positive endometrial, ovarian, and breast security profile [39, 40].

A phase III, multi-centre, double-blind, randomised, controlled trial was formulated with the sole purpose of assessing the effectiveness of bazedoxifene in fracture prevention. The trial looked at 7,492 healthy postmenopausal women presenting with osteoporosis both with or without prevalent vertebral fractures. The women were randomly assigned to 20 or 40mg per day of bazedoxifene, 60mg of raloxifene, or to a placebo plus 1200mg of calcium and 400IU of vitamin D. The primary outcome was the occurrence of new vertebral fractures following a three-year treatment period. Secondary indicators included clinical vertebral fractures, worsening of vertebral fractures, non-vertebral fractures, breast cancer incidence, and variations in height. Both bazedoxifene 20 and 40mg reduced the occurrence of vertebral fractures to a similar extent as raloxifene versus the placebo. The occurrence at 36 months of new vertebral fractures was 2.3%, 2.5%, 2.3%, and 4.1% in the bazedoxifene 20mg, bazedoxifene 40mg, raloxifene 60mg, and placebo cohorts, respectively, with a distinct lowering of the relative incidence for new vertebral fractures of 42%, 37%, and 42%, respectively, versus placebo. There was no overall impact on non-vertebral fractures, with incidence rates of 5.7% and 5.6% for the bazedoxifene 20 and 40mg cohorts, respectively, versus 5.9% for the raloxifene cohort and 6.3% for the placebo cohort. Nevertheless, in a later review of women with elevated fracture risk (poor femoral neck T-score and multiple vertebral fractures, n=1,772), bazedoxifene 20mg reduced the incidence of non-vertebral fracture by 50% and 44% reduction relative to the placebo (HR=0.50; 95% CI: 0.28–0.90; p=0.02) and raloxifene 60mg (HR=0.56; 95% CI: 0.31–1.01; p=0.05), respectively [41].

2.3.2.3. *Safety*

Miller et al. demonstrated that deep venous thromboembolism was uncommon with bazedoxifene (0% to 0.6% with varying dosage levels after two years) and similar to the placebo (0.3%). The rate of occurrence and the intensity of hot flushes were comparable with raloxifene, but slightly elevated versus placebo [40]. In the trial by Silverman et al., leg cramps (10.9% to 11.7% with varying dosage after three years) and deep venous thromboembolism (0.4% to 0.5% with varying dosage after three years) were decidedly more prevalent with bazedoxifene compared with the placebo (8.2% for leg cramps and 0.2% for deep venous thromboembolism), while fibrocystic breast disease was markedly less frequent. No distinction in risk levels between bazedoxifene and placebo was noted for myocardial infarction, strokes (ischemic or hemorraghic), or retinal vein thrombosis [40-43].

We can conclude that bazedoxifene appears to have improved selectivity in contrast with other SERMs. The impact of bazedoxifene on the skeleton is not dissimilar to raloxifene, and bazedoxifene may be employed in the same way as raloxifene. The usefulness of bazedoxifene possibly lies in its risk profile being distinct to that of raloxifene, particularly with regards to uterine safety, and bazedoxifene may therefore present another option for the prevention and treatment of osteoporosis.

2.3.3. *Lasofoxifene*

Lasofoxifene is a powerful third-generation SERM. It has a distinct structure compared to first- and second-generation SERMs (raloxifene, tamoxifen and clomiphene or idoxifene). Lasofoxifene displays powerful estrogenic and anti-estrogenic activity in vitro and in vivo, targeting any areas with estrogens receptors, including bone, uterus, breast, blood vessels, and liver. Lasofoxifene has been analysed in postmenopausal women with regards to the prevention and treatment of osteoporosis. Security and tolerance levels of lasofoxifene is similar to that of raloxifene, however nonadherence rates as a result of adverse events are greater with lasofoxifene. Despite these indications, results demonstrate that lasofoxifene treatment may lead to greater endometrial thickness versus the placebo, despite there being no evidence of an elevated incidence of endometrial hyperplasia or cancer.

The PEARL study, a three-year pivotal fracture study, showed that lasofoxifene elevated lumbar spine and femoral neck BMD by approximately 3%. Furthermore, vertebral fractures saw a decrease of 42%, and non-vertebral fractures of 27%, with a decrease in markers of bone turnover. Nevertheless, lasofoxifene did not reduce the risk of hip fractures [43].

2.4. Bisphosphonates

2.4.1. Analysis and mode of action

Bisphosphonates are a member of a class of antiresorptive agents whose antifracture action is well-documented through randomised controlled studies. There have been no studies to compare different bisphosphonates, a fact which has prevented the identification of a definite order of effectiveness for treatment.

Bisphosphonates lower fracture risk as a result of its inhibitory action of osteoclasts, which enables the osteoblasts to synthesize bone in the resorption spaces and some bone lacunae. This produces an augmentation in bone mass. However, the bisphosphonates also increase bone quality, by conserving the bone architecture, as demonstrated in studies which have analysed the biopsies of treated patients and control subjects.

Bisphosphonates comprise pyrophosphate analogs in which the central oxygen has been replaced by a carbon atom and two side chains (R1 and R2). Two phosphate chains are vital to enable the drug to bind to bone and to have an antiresorptive effect.

2.4.2. Etidronate

Etidronate was the original bisphosphonate used in osteoporosis therapy. It is no longer used in current practice. Its greatest asset is most likely its cost. It augments bone mass in the spine and femur and lowers the risk of vertebral fractures, however it has not demonstrated a reduction in the incidence of femoral fractures [44,45].

2.4.3. Clodronate

Clodronate has been deployed in postmenopausal osteoporosis therapy in oral and intravenous treatments. The trials indicate that it reduces the risk of bone loss in the vertebral spine in comparison to control subjects, and it presents similar results to estrogens after two years. In a six-year long study, it was also demonstrated to lower the incidence rate of vertebral fractures. McCloskey et al. carried out a three-year, double-blind, controlled study to observe the impact of oral clodronate (800mg per day) on fracture rates. In this study, clodronate was linked with a distinct improvement in the mean lumbar spine and hip BMD. Furthermore, it significantly lowered the risk of vertebral fracture (relative risk, 0,54; 95% CI, 0,37-0,80; $p<0,0001$). Despite these outcomes, subsequent to the introduction of powerful nitrogen bisphosphonates, the first-generation bisphosphonates have been reduced to a therapy of last resort [46].

2.4.4. Alendronate (alendronic acid)

Alendronate is one of the most commonly deployed bisphosphonates. It augments vertebral bone mass approximately 6-8% and 3-6% at the hip in postmenopausal osteoporotic women after a three-year treatment. It demonstrates a reduction in vertebral and non-vertebral fractures of around 50% in this time period. In male osteoporosis, it has demonstrated improvements in bone mass of 5% after two years of treatment.

Alendronate is given orally, in doses of 70mg/week, fasting with 200 ml of water. The patient is prohibited from consuming solids or liquids for 30 minutes after treatment and must remain standing for this time.

The decisive study of alendronate, the FIT (Fracture Intervention Trial), demonstrated that the incidence of clinical fracture was reduced for the alendronate cohort compared to the control cohort (139 (13.6%) versus 183 (18.2%); relative hazard=0.72 (0.58-0.90)). The corresponding risk of hip and wrist fracture for the alendronate cohort when compared to the placebo cohort were 0.49 (0.23-0.99) and 0.52 (0.31-0.87) [47]. Ensrud et al. provided an assessment of a subset of FIT subjects who were patients with an elevated risk of fracture. The outcomes of this analysis demonstrate a decisive 47% lowering of the risk of new vertebral fractures in the alendronate cohort when set against the control cohort. A number of other papers have been generated from the FIT study, addressing multiple symptomatic fractures, bone mineral density, biochemical markers of formation and resorption, fracture prevention in osteopenic women, impact of alendronate continuation versus discontinuation, and the impact on women who lost bone over the course of treatment [48-51].

We can conclude that alendronate is a well-tolerated, secure and efficacious treatment method for postmenopausal osteoporosis, male osteoporosis, and glucocorticoid induced osteoporosis (GIOP).

2.4.5. Risedronate

This treatment has been proven to improve bone mass in spine and hip and to considerably lower the incidence of fracture in postmenopausal women. Treatment of postmenopausal women with osteoporosis with risedronate over a three-year period has produced a reduction in the risk of vertebral fractures in roughly 50% and non-vertebral fractures in 39% of subjects. At the hip, the fracture reduction rate is between 40 and 60%. After a five-year period, the outcomes are comparable. The treatment has demonstrated its anti-fracture efficacy after a six-month course. In other trials it has been proven that this reduction in risk was still present following a seven-year period of treatment, and was accompanied by a positive security profile. One of the principal studies of risedronate [52] looked at 5,445 women aged 70 to 79 years with osteoporosis (T-score at the femoral neck greater than -4 SD below the mean or lower than -3 plus a non-skeletal risk factor for hip fracture, such as poor gait or a tendency to fall) and 3,886 women aged at least 80 years with a minimum of one non-skeletal risk factor for hip fracture or poor BMD at the femoral neck (T-score below -4 or below -3 plus a hip-axis length of 11.1cm or greater). The subjects were given a treatment at random of either oral risedronate (2.5 or 5.0mg per day) or a placebo, over a three-year period. The outcomes indicated that the risk of hip fracture among subjects given risedronate was 2.8%, versus 3.9% among those given the placebo (relative risk, 0.7; 95% CI, 0.6 to 0.9; p=0.02). In the cohort of women with osteoporosis (70 to 79 years old), the risk of hip fracture among subjects given risedronate was 1.9%, versus 3.2% among subjects given the placebo (relative risk, 0.6; 95% CI,

0.4 to 0.9; p=0.009). In the cohort of subjects chosen principally for non-skeletal risk factors (those at least 80 years old), the risk of hip fracture was 4.2% for subjects given risedronate and 5.1% for those given the placebo (p=0.35) [52].

To assess the impact on vertebral fracture risk, Reginster et al. carried out a randomised, double-blind, controlled trial to evaluate the effectiveness and security of risedronate for reducing the risk of vertebral fractures in postmenopausal women with established osteoporosis. The trial was carried out at 80 locations in Europe and Australia. In total, 1,226 postmenopausal women with two or more prevalent vertebral fractures were given risedronate 2.5mg or 5mg per day or a placebo. Whilst the trial was carried out over three years, the 2.5mg cohort was ended by protocol amendment after two years. Risedronate 5mg lowered the incidence of new vertebral fractures by 49% over three years in comparison with the placebo (p<0.001). A distinct decrease of 61% was witnessed over the initial year alone (p=0.001). The decreased incidence of fracture was comparable in both cohorts after two years. The incidences of non-vertebral fracture saw a decrease of 33% in relation to the placebo figures over three years (p=0.06). Risedronate produced a distinct elevation in BMD at the spine and hip within a six-month period. We can conclude that risedronate 5mg was an efficacious and well-tolerated treatment for severe postmenopausal osteoporosis, decreasing the risk of vertebral fractures and increasing bone density in women with chronic osteoporosis [53].

2.4.6. Ibandronate

In trials lasting three years, ibandronate has been proven to decrease the risk of vertebral fractures (52%) and improve vertebral BMD (6.5%) whilst not having a substantial negative impact on bone histology. It has also shown to be very efficacious in reducing bone loss in GIOP (glucocorticoid induced osteoporosis). In women with severe osteoporosis T scores (<-3), it decreases the risk of non-vertebral fractures up to 69% [54].

Randomised clinical studies such as MOPS (Monthly Oral Pilot Study) or MOBILE (Monthly Oral Ibandronate in Ladies) have indicated that the ibandronate monthly dosage is just as efficacious and safe as the daily dosage. Amongst the general population of the pivotal trial (BONE, Oral Ibandronate Osteoporosis Vertebral Fracture Trial in North America and Europe), the likelihood of adverse incidents of the gastrointestinal tract in both the daily and the intermittent treatment cohorts was similar to the control cohort. Dyspepsia was the only adverse incident with a marginally greater rate in subjects undergoing therapy with ibandronate [55].

2.4.7. Zoledronate (zoledronic acid)

Zoledronic acid is a third-generation bisphosphonate. It is roughly as powerful as alendronate, risedronate and ibandronate, however the application of this drug intravenously prevents any negative impact and in fact augments the bioavailability, whilst also improving compliance to 100%.

The HORIZON trial (Health Outcomes and Reduced Incidence with Zoledonic Acid Once Yearly Pivotal Fracture Trial) was a global, multi-centre, double-blind, controlled study of postmenopausal women with osteoporosis, whose goal was to demonstrate the increase efficacy of intravenous zoledronic acid 5mg compared with a control. Subjects presented with densitometric osteoporosis or densitometric osteopenia with a minimum of 2 mild to moderate vertebral fractures [56]. Over 7,700 women were involved in the trial and were monitored over a three-year period; particular scrutiny was made of new fractures, bone remodeling biochemical markers and densitometric developments. On completion of the trial, subjects that had been treated with zoledronic acid presented a decrease in the vertebral fracture risk of 70%. The decrease was comparable for the first two years of the trial, varying from 60% to 71%. In addition, subjects given zoledronate presented a decrease of 41% in hip fracture incidence and 25% in non-vertebral fracture incidence. The outcomes of bone density and biochemical bone remodeling markers were also markedly improved for the cohort given zoledronic acid. Furthermore, bone mineral density was elevated to over 6% in the lumbar spine and total hip, and to over 5% in the femoral neck. The biochemical markers of bone remodeling, after the initial transfusion of zoledronic acid, decreased significantly as anticipated, and stayed stable throughout the remainder of the trial [57].

Many subjects experienced adverse effects over the course of the trial, with a greater occurrence of these in the zoledronate cohort. This variance was explained by post-infusion syndrome, which commonly manifested itself 24-48 hours after the zoledronic acid infusion and dissipated three days after infusion. The syndrome presented with mild fever, myalgias, flu-like symptoms, headache and/or arthralgias and was dissipated with analgesic, non-steroid anti-inflammatory drugs or acetaminophen. A few subjects presented with passing renal function deterioration 9 to 11 days post-infusion, however these instances were of no clinical transcendence [57].

Perhaps the most significant conclusion in relation to zoledronate therapy is the 28% decrease in mortality of any cause, which was demonstrated in a cohort of over 2,000 subjects with femur fracture [56].

We can conclude that zoledronate therapy is extremely efficacious in the reduction of vertebral, non-vertebral and hip fractures. It reduces mortality, independent of the cause, following a femur fracture.Moreover, it is a low-risk therapy that avoids the gastrointestinal adverse events and high nonadherence rates that are commonly encountered with other bisphosphonates, but it should be dispensed and regulated with great caution when treating individuals with severe renal function impairment.

2.4.8. Safety of bisphosphonates

This class of treatments is usually well-tolerated, provided that they are administered carefully and that patients adhere to the instructions for their use. Esophageal ulcerations been encountered in situations where these treatments are given orally and on a daily basis. They must not be given to patients with gastric or esophageal ulcerations, or to patients with pyrosis (heartburn) which requires treatment. They must not be administered to pregnant women, or to individuals with chronic renal impairment. The intravenous bisphosphonates normally give rise to acute phase reactions with fever, arthromyalgia and flu-like symptoms that commonly dissipate before the second dosage and which can be mitigated by giving acetaminophen or ibuprofen concurrently. Hypocalcaemia can present more frequently, so it is advisable to give calcium and vitamin D concurrently. The renal function has to be regulated both prior to and following treatments of intravenous bisphosphonates.

The avascular necrosis of the jaw, also called osteonecrosis of the jaw, is a condition which has concerned many practitioners since Marx identified it for the first time in 2003 and it ought to be outlined more completely in another chapter [58].

2.4.9. Long-term impact of bisphosphonate therapies: Atypical hip fractures

Research linking atypical fractures of the femur with longstanding treatments of bisphosphonates caused the American Society for Bone and Mineral Research (ASBMR) to launch an enquiry to consider the important queries raised by the conclusions of this research. The enquiry's committee identified both major and minor features of incomplete and complete atypical femoral fractures and advised that all significant features, including their location in the subtrochanteric region and femoral shaft, transverse or short oblique orientation, little or no associated trauma, a medial spike when the fracture is complete, and lack of comminution, be discernible in order to designate a femoral fracture as atypical. Minor features include the fracture's relationship with cortical thickening, a periosteal reaction of the lateral cortex, prodromal pain, bilaterality, delayed healing, co-morbid conditions, and concurrent drug usage, including bisphosphonates, other antiresorptive agents, glucocorticoids, and proton pump inhibitors. On the strength of published and unpublished information and the wide application of bisphosphonates, the occurrence of atypical femoral fractures linked with bisphosphonate use for osteoporosis seems to be decidedly uncommon, especially in relation to the extent to which vertebral, hip, and other fractures are in turn prevented. Moreover, a causal link between bisphosphonates and atypical fractures has not been demonstrated. Nevertheless, new investigations infer that the incidence rate increases with longer periods of therapy, and there is a feeling of unease that a lack of understanding and underreporting could be hiding the true extent of the issue.

A 2008 trial of 12,777 Swedish women aged 55 years or more with a fracture of the femur was made public recently. Radiographs of 1,234 of 1,271 women presenting a subtrochanteric or shaft fracture were analysed. Fifty-nine subjects with atypical fractures were isolated. The relative and absolute incidence of atypical fractures linked with bisphosphonate treatment was calculated using a national cohort analysis. The 59 subjects were also subject to a comparison with 263 control subjects who presented typical subtrochanteric or shaft fractures. The cohort analysis indicated an age-adjusted proportional risk of atypical fracture of 47.3. The rise in global risk was 5 instances per 10,000 patient-years. In total, 78% of the fractured patients and 10% of the controls had been given bisphosphonates (multivariable-adjusted odds ratio of 33.3). The incidence level was independent of coexisting ailments. Following cessation of treatment, the incidence level was reduced by 70% per year from the time of last use (odds ratio, 0.28; 95% CI, 0.21 to 0.38) [59].

2.5. Biological agents

Conditions that give rise to bone loss, like osteoporosis, are caused by the imbalance in the cycles of bone remodeling favouring bone resorption. The receptor activator of the nuclear factor kB (RANK), and its ligand (RANKL) are critical for the differentiation, activation and survival of osteoclasts and, as a result are the most simple intermediary in the regulating of bone remodeling (Burgess et al.1999). It has been proven that the signaling of the RANKL is inherent to the pathophysiology of many bone loss conditions, such as primary and many secondary forms of osteoporosis.

2.5.1. Denosumab

Denosumab is a fully human monoclonal IgG2 antibody to RANKL that imitates the effects of osteoprotegerine (OPG), endogenous inhibitor of RANKL that blocks bone resorption.

Comercial denosumab is sold as a sterile, uncolored solution administered via subcutaneous injection.

2.5.1.1. Denosumab in human clinical studies

Data is accessible from more than 50 clinical studies in healthy adults and patients with osteoporosis, bone loss linked with hormone-ablation treatments, rheumatoid arthritis, advanced cancer (multiple myeloma and advanced malignancies that involve bone and giant cell tumor of the bone collected since June 2001).

In the *Denosumab Fortifies Bone Density* (DEFEND) trial, a phase III, randomised, controlled trial of 332 postmenopausal women with osteopenia sorted by the length of menopause (<5 years, >5 years), denosumab showed a distinctive rise in lumbar BMD (6.5%) at the two-year point, in relation to the control (-0.6%). It also raised BMD in other sites including total hip, distal third of the radius, and whole body (p>0.001) in the two cohorts. The rate of side effects was comparable between the control cohort and the denosumab cohort [60].

In a comparative clinical study, the DECIDE (*Determining Efficacy: Comparison of Initiating Denosumab vs. Alendronate*) trial of 1,189 postmenopausal women with low BMD (T-score: ≤-2 SD), subjects were randomly allocated 1:1 to two groups, one to be given subcutaneous denosumab (60mg per 6 months) plus an oral alendronate placebo weekly or oral alendronate weekly (70mg) plus a subcutaneous denosumab placebo injection every 6 months. Denosumab raised total hip BMD in relation to alendronate (3.5% versus 2.5%, p<0.00001). A more significant increase in BMD could be witnessed with denosumab than with alendronate in other locations, as in the trochanter (4.5% vs. 3.5%), distal radius (1.1% versus 0.6%), lumbar spine (5.3% versus 4.2%) and femoral neck (2.2% versus 1.6%); p<0.0003. The security profile was comparable for the two cohorts. No subject in the trial developed antibodies in reaction to denosumab [61].

Another phase III, multi-centre, double-blind trial, named STAND (*Study of transitioning from Alendronate to Denosumab*) was carried out to assess the impact of denosumab in subjects who were undergoing alendronate treatment. Five hundred and four postmenopausal women ≥ 55 years old with a BMD T-score of <-2.0 and >-4 SD, who were taking weekly oral alendronate for a minimum of six months, were randomly assigned to the treatment for 44±33 months. Alterations to BMD and bone biochemical markers were assessed. After a year, the cohort taking denosumab (and had been given alendronate before the trial) presented a markedly elevated total hip BMD in comparison with the cohort which continued to take alendronate (1.9% versus 1.05%; $p<0.00012$). Markedly elevated BMD readings with denosumab in comparison with alendronate were also noted after one year at the lumbar spine, femoral neck, and distal radius (all $p<0.0125$). The side effects and serious side effects were comparable in both cohorts [62].

Lastly, the principal phase III study, the FREEDOM (*Fracture Reduction Evaluation of Denosumab in Osteoporosis every 6 Months*) study, involved 7,868 postmenopausal women with osteoporosis and a BMD T-score between <-2.0 and >-4 SD and assessed the effectiveness in fracture reduction of denosumab. Subjects were given 60mg subcutaneous denosumab or placebo every six months for three years. Approximately 23% of the subjects had experienced a prior vertebral fracture. The trial's retention rate of subjects was 83%. The decrease in relative risk of fracture was 68% (2.3% versus 7.2%; $p<0.0001$) for vertebral fractures, 20% (6.5% versus 8.0%) for non-vertebral fractures and 40% (0.7% versus 1.2%) for hip fractures. In comparison to patients in the control cohort, patients in the denosumab cohort saw a proportional elevation of 9.2% in bone mineral density at the lumbar spine and 6.0% at the total hip at three years. No distinctive dissimilarities were apparent between patients who were given denosumab and those who were given a placebo in the overall rate of side effects, serious side effects, or nonadherence to the trial as a result of side effects. No instances of osteonecrosis of the jaw were found in either cohort during this decisive study (Cummings et al. 2009). Lastly, the positive effects of denosumab therapy were generally discernible following the first treatment and remained so over the course of up to eight years of denosumab therapy in an open-ended extension trial [63].

We can conclude that denosumab provides an extremely efficacious substitute for osteoporosis therapy through the reduction of bone resorption and the elevation of bone mineral density via the inhibition of RANKL. A distinct benefit of denosumab is its route of administration and dosage. A subcutaneous injection every 6 months is comparatively free of discomfort and improves the therapy retention levels.

3. Anabolic agents

3.1. Fluoride

A series of observations were published indicating a low occurrence of fracture in subjects residing in locations with elevated fluoride levels. Fluoride was first employed in osteoporosis therapy in 1961. It was authorised for the prevention of osteoporosis in several European countried, but was never given authorisation by the American Federal Drug Administration (FDA) [64,65].

The outcomes of studies into the impact of fluoride on the reduction of fracture risk are ambiguous. Some trials have shown a reduction in the risk of vertebral fractures under monofluorophosphate, or sodium fluoride treatment, whereas other trials, giving patients the same preparations and dosage, did not. In addition, one meta-analysis extends these investigations and identifies an elevated fracture risk with increasing dosages after four years [66-68]. As a result, fluoride is not employed in the treatment of osteoporosis any longer.

3.2. Teriparatide (1-34 parathohormone)

Within the range of treatment options available, teriparatide or recombinant human PTH (1-34), has a significant role to play. It is a member of the group of anabolic bone-forming drugs rather than the anti-resorptive or catabolic group. It is a catalyst for fresh bone formation by accelerating bone turnover in favour of formation. Teriparatide therapy improves trabecular connectivity and cortical bone thickness [69] and augments the mechanical properties of bone causing a marked reduction in vertebral and non-vertebral fractures in postmenopausal women with osteoporosis, male osteoporosis and corticosteroid-induced osteoporosis [70]. For this reason its application is deemed to be suitable mostly for individuals at high risk of fracture and for those for whom other drugs have been unsuccessful [71].

The original indication for teriparatide first made public was the treatment of established osteoporosis in postmenopausal women. Amongst the varying trials which have been carried out on this treatment, the FPT (Fracture Prevention Trial) is the most significant. It assessed teriparatide at dosages of 20 or 40μg/day in controlled conditions in 1,637 postmenopausal women with vertebral fractures. Subjects taking teriparatide presented a marked decrease in the rate of fresh vertebral and non-vertebral fractures. They also experienced elevated lumbar and femoral neck bone density. Whilst the 40μg/day dose had a greater impact on BMD, the risk of fracture did not vary to any marked extent between the two dosage levels, while the higher dosage was less tolerated (11% nonretention due to adverse events with 40μg/day compared with 6% with 20 μg/day or with the placebo). The dosage of 20μg/day presented a decreased risk of vertebral fracture of 65% and a decreased risk of non-hip non-vertebral fracture risk reduction of 35%. This trial was originally supposed to run over a 36-month period, but it was terminated when subjects had undergone on average 21 months of treatment for safety reasons following osteosarcomas witnessed in rats during drug toxicity trials [72]. In other trials it transpired nevertheless that this effect presented only in juvenile rats given with elevated doses of PTH [73]. In addition, no instances of osteosarcomas have been noted in humans.

A subset of subjects were monitored for a maximum of 18 months following the termination of the therapy. This subset, which had been given teriparatide, demonstrated an enduring 40% decrease in vertebral fracture risk at 18 months versus the control sample. These outcomes indicate that the drug's positive impact on the rate of non-vertebral fractures continues beyond the termination of treatment [74].

3.2.1. Combination therapy: Teriparatide plus antiresorptives.

Despite bisphosphonates being the current benchmark for the treatment of osteoporosis, several studies exist that have assessed whether the combination of teriparatide and BP can produce a positive impact. The trials indicate that, if both treatments are given at the same time, bisphosphonates reduce rather than increase the anabolic action of teriparatide [75].

Combined teriparatide and denosumab, on the other hand, improves spine and hip BMD to a greater extent than either treatment does when administered in isolation. In the DATA-HRpQCT study, subjects underwent high-resolution peripheral QCT assessments at the distal tibia and radius (postmenopausal osteoporotic women randomly assigned to take teriparatide 20μg daily (n=31), denosumab 60mg every 6 months (n=33), or both (n=30) for 12 months). In the teriparatide cohort, the overall volumetric BMD (vBMD) did not vary at either anatomic location but was improved in both other cohorts at both locations. The elevated vBMD at the tibia showed an increase in the combination cohort (3.1±2.2%) compared with either the denosumab (2.2±1.9%) or teriparatide cohort (-0.3±1.9%) ($p<0.02$). Cortical vBMD was reduced by 1.6±1.9% at the tibia and by 0.9±2.8% at the radius in the teriparatide cohort whilst it was elevated in both other cohorts at both anatomic locations. Tibia cortical vBMD saw greater increases in the combination cohort (1.5±1.5%) than in the other two cohorts ($p<0.04$ for both comparisons). Cortical thickness was not affected in the teriparatide cohort, but was elevated in the other cohorts. Elevations in cortical thickness at the tibia was more marked in the combination cohort (5.4±3.9%) than the other cohorts ($p<0.01$ for both comparisons). In the teriparatide cohort, radial cortical porosity was raised by 20.9±37.6% and by 5.6±9.9% at the tibia but was not affected in the other two cohorts. Bone stiffness and failure load, as calculated through finite element analysis, was not affected in the teriparatide cohort but was elevated in the other two cohorts at both locations. These results suggest that the application of denosumab combined with teriparatide has a positive impact on HR-pQCT indices of bone quality to a greater extent than either treatment in isolation and may be of significant clinical benefit in the management of postmenopausal osteoporosis [76].

3.2.2. Teriparatide in individuals formerly given antiresorptives

The EUROFORS study was a prospective, open-label, randomised study of 865 postmenopausal women with established osteoporosis and aimed to assess a variety of consecutive applications of teriparatide over a two-year period. Subjects were split into several subsets based on their former therapies. The outcomes of the BMD variations and biochemical markers of bone formation indicated that the application of teriparatide has a beneficial impact on bone mass and osteoblast function in postmenopausal women with established osteoporosis whatever the extent or type of former long-term exposure to antiresorptive treatments has been.

The length of the antiresorptive treatment and the length of pause in treatment between the former therapy and the teriparatide had no impact on BMD levels at any anatomic location. The skeletal reaction at the lumbar spine was comparable among former antiresorptive treatment cohorts at every point in time over the course of the trial, however subjects who had previously been given etidronate presented a greater increase, most likely a factor of its poorer anti-remodeling action. At six months, overall hip and femoral neck BMD showed a marked reduction in the former alendronate subset, and total hip BMD showed a marked reduction in the former risedronate subset. Overall hip and femoral neck BMD was statistically reduced from baseline in all other subsets at the six-month point. Nevertheless, this short-term reduction was contradicted over longer-term teriparatide therapy. All subsets demonstrated a numerically distinctive rise in BMD versus baseline after 18 and 24 months of therapy, and without variations between the cohorts at any point in the trial [77].

3.2.3. Sequential treatment

In a further non-randomised trial, 59 postmenopausal women with osteoporosis formerly given raloxifene or alendronate over an 18-36 month period, were treated with teriparatide over 18 months. Variations in BMD and bone-turnover markers were analysed. Subjects who had formerly been given alendronate saw a delayed rise in bone-turnover markers with results more than a third lower than those of subjects who had formerly been given raloxifene. Over the initial six-month period there were marked variations in the rise in BMD at the lumbar spine and hip. Subjects formerly given raloxifene saw more significant rises in BMD at the two sites. After 18 months of therapy marked variations continued in the lumbar spine, with greater improvement in subjects previously given raloxifene, however the variations in the hip were not as decisive. This proves that this application of teriparatide augments bone turnover in subjects formerly given raloxifene or alendronate, and that this improvement comes sooner and is more significant with the raloxifene pretreatment cohort [78].

3.2.4. Corticosteroid-induced osteoporosis and male osteoporosis

Studies have also been published which demonstrate the effectiveness of teriparatide in the management of GIOP. In a randomised, double-blind study, 428 subjects both male and female from 22 to 89 years old, who had been given corticosteroids for a minimum of three months were randomly assigned to be treated with either alendronate 10mg/day or teriparatide 20μg/day over an 18 month period. After a year, the overall femur BMD was greater in the teriparatide cohort and on termination of the trial there were fewer vertebral fractures in the teriparatide cohort [79].

Teriparatide has also been employed as a treatment in men with osteoporosis. The trial analysed results from men with idiopathic or secondary osteoporosis being treated with teriparatide in comparison with a control group. The trial indicated elevated results, independent of gonadal status and other influential elements in the teriparatide cohort [80].

3.2.5. Adverse Effects

Overall, teriparatide (recombinant human PTH (1-34)) injections are well-tolerated. It disappears from the bloodstream in less than four hours following subcutaneous administration. Injections on a daily basis are required and a passing reddening at the injection site has been observed. Headache and nausea have been noted in under 10% of patients treated with a daily dose of 20μg. Mild, early, short-term hypercalcemia can transpire, but severe hypercalcemia is uncommon. Higher levels of urinary calcium (up 30μg per day) and serum uric acid concentrations (up 13%) are witnessed, however these do not seem to have clinical ramifications.

We can conclude that teriparatide is an appropriate and effective drug for the management of osteoporosis. It is efficacious in addressing a variety of clinical conditions, e.g. male osteoporosis or corticosteroid-induced osteoporosis.

3.3. 1-84 Parathormone

Intact PTH (PTH 1-84) has been reported to have a beneficial impact on bone micro-architecture and to reduce incidence of fresh fractures as a result of its bone-forming mode of action [81].

PTH 1-84 is not procurable any more due to the withdrawal of its marketing licence at the behest of the regulating authority.

4. Dual action agents

4.1. Strontium ranelate

The possible clinical applications of strontium were revealed in approximately 1940, when strontium-89 was deployed as an analgesic treatment for bone metastases caused by prostate cancer [82,83].

In-vitro, strontium ranelate augments collagen and non-collagen protein synthesis through mature osteoblasts. The bone-forming action has been demonstrated by the higher levels of replication amongst pre-osteoblastic cells. This catalytic action on the duplication of pre-osteoblastic cells and the higher levels of collagen and non-collagen proteins have caused strontium ranelate to be regarded as a dual effect bone agent, because it does not simply reduce resorption [84]. The principal tool that can determine bone resorption at a molecular level is the RANK/RNAKL/OPG system outlined above. Solutions of 0.1mM to 2nM of strontium ranelate reduce the capacity of human osteoblasts to cause osteoclast differentiation, by reducing expression of mRNA of RANK-L and boosting mRNA expression of OPG, as reported in the trials carried out by Brennan et al. in 2006 [85, 86].

4.1.1. Impact of Strontium ranelate in fracture reduction

Studies have shown that the chemical properties of strontium ranelate cause the, densitometric values of subjects given the compound to be greater than the true values. Complex mathematical formulas exist to cut out the statistical impact of this from the DMO value, however it is more straightforward and sufficiently accurate to assume instead that half of the DMO achieved in the first year of therapy with strontium ranelate is a result of elevations in BMD and the remainder is a result of the basis caused by the heavier strontium measured by the DXA [87].

Information from the SOTI (Spinal Osteoporosis Therapeutic Intervention) study and the TROPOS (Treatment of Peripheral Osteoporosis) study looked at 1,649 postmenopausal subjects (SOTI trial) and 5,091 subjects (TROPOS trial) [88,89]. The initial three-year outcomes demonstrated a decrease in vertebral fractures of 41% with a NNT of 9. Moreover, an im-

http://dx.doi.org/10.5772/59469

provement in BMD of 12.7% was recorded. The decrease in vertebral fractures at the end of the four- and five-year periods was 33% and 24% respectively. In relation to non-vertebral fractures, the reduction in the relative incidence of fracture with strontium ranelate was 16% at the end of the three-year period and 15% at the end of the five-year period. A later assessment of these results in a subset of 1,977 subjects with high fracture risk (≥74 years old and a T-score of ≤-2.4) indicated a decrease in the incidence of vertebral fracture of 36% at the end of the three-year period and 43% at the end of the five-year period [87, 90].

4.1.2. Security

Strontium ranelate was deployed in a widespread manner across Europe up to February 2014, when the European Medicines Agency (EMA) advised that the use of the drug be limited to cases which cannot use other treatments approved for osteoporosis, and that subjects with high risk for ischemic cardiac disorders should be excluded from this treatment option. This decision was grounded in a study carried out by the Pharmacovigilance Risk Assessment Committee (PRAC) that highlighted doubts about cardiovascular security which went beyond the risk, already known, of venous thromboembolism. On the basis of the PRAC analysis, an elevated incidence of serious cardiac disorders (including myocardial infarction) was pinpointed and steps were put forward to minimize the risk, specifically targeting the highlighted issue, in April 2013.

5. Overview of current treatments

As set out in this review, there are several treatment options for osteoporosis. Unfortunately the choices are more restricted in daily clinical practice as treatments have been removed or their use restricted. Table 2 provides a summary of those treatments currently available to practitioners.

Drug	Indications (in OP)	Dose in OP	Route	Bone resorption	Bone formation	Vertebral fractures	Non-vertebral fractures	Hip fractures
Raloxifene	Postmenopausal OP	60 mg/d	Oral	↓↓	↓↓	+	±	Ø
Bazedoxifene	Postmenopausal OP	20 mg/d	Oral	↓↓	↓↓	+	±	Ø
Alendronate	Postmenopausal OP	70 mg/w	Oral	↓↓↓	↓↓↓	+	+	+
Risedronate	Postmenopausal and Male OP	35 mg/w	Oral	↓↓↓	↓↓↓	+	+	+
Ibandronate	Postmenopausal OP	150mg/m	Oral	↓↓↓	↓↓↓	+	±	Ø
Zoledronate	Postmenopausal, Male and GC OP	5 mg/year	IV	↓↓↓	↓↓↓	+	+	+
Denosumab	Postmenopausal and Male OP	60mg/6m	SC	↓↓↓	↓	+	+	+
Teriparatide	Postmenopausal, Male and GC OP	20μg/d	SC	↑↑	↑↑↑	+	+	Ø
Strontium Ranelate	Postmenopausal and Male OP	2g/d	Oral	↓	↑	+	+	±

Table 2. Current available osteoporosis therapies

6. Future treatment options

6.1. Cathepsine K (CatK) inhibitors

Cathepsin K is expressed in the main in osteoclasts and a variety of other multinucleated cells including giant foreign body cells and Langhans cells. To a lesser extent it is present in macrophages, synovial fibroblasts, and fibroblasts at sites of wound repair or inflammation, chondrocytes, various epithelial cells of the human fetus, adult lung airway epithelium, thyroid epithelium, and potentially in low levels within smooth muscle cells. When the enzyme has been synthesised, it is separated into lysosomes and can be introduced into the extracellular environment. It is introduced particularly into the resorption lacuna below actively resorbing osteclasts where it is causes the degradation of the collagen type I dominated organic bone matrix. Thus, in a similar manner to pycnoidisostosis, removal of cathepsin K from osteoclasts prevents bone resorption. Inhibitors of cathepsin K are reported to have a less significant impact on osteoclast–osteoblast interaction, causing a lower inhibition of bone formation than available bisphosphonate antiresorptive drugs. Human cathepsin K inhibitors have been proven to stop bone loss in ovariectomized mice without reducing the anabolic effeciveness of parathyroid hormone (PTH) [91].

Whilst no CatK inhibitor is licensed for osteoporosis treatment or prevention at the present time, trials of three CatK inhibitors for the management of osteoporosis have been published: balicatib, relacatib, and odanacatib.

6.1.1. Balicatib

Balicatib is extremely selective for CatK in enzyme potency tests but has a reduced selectivity in living tissue. Clinical trials of balicatib have shown elevated BMD in postmenopausal women, but the drug was linked with cutaneous adverse effects. The first presentation of the efficacy of cathepsin K inhibitors on human bone density was witnessed with balicatib. This study, released by Adami et al. at an ASBMR meeting in 2009 (Denver, CO, USA), was a multi-centre, randomised, controlled, 12 month, dose-range identifying trial of 675 postmenopausal subjects with lumbar spine T-score less than 2.0. In the cohort treated with 50mg of balicatib daily, markers of bone resorption were reduced by over 55% with no reduction in markers of bone formation (osteocalcin, bone-specific alkaline phosphatase and N-terminal propeptide of type I collagen). The lumbar spine BMD was elevated 4.46%, that of the total hip was elevated 2.25%. Cutaneous reactions, including pruritus and morphea-like alterations, were observed in a low number of subjects. In a limited Japanese study, intact PTH levels were demonstrated to be elevated by 50% with balicatib treatment [92].

6.1.2. Relacatib

Relacatib is a powerful but nonselective inhibitor of cathepsins K, L, V, and S for which no clinical data in humans has been made public. The use of relacatib with ovariectomized and control monkeys caused an acute and rapid decrease in bone markers, and the impact of this lasted for a maximum of 48 hours, according to the dosage administered [93].

On the basis of the adverse effects, especially the cutaneous reactions, the production of all cathepsin K inhibitor drugs has been discontinued or put on hold, with the exception of odanacatib and, at present, ONO 5334

6.1.3. Odanacatib

Odanacatib is a potent, selective inhibitor with an ability to inhibit cathepsin K in osteoclasts [91].

Two trials have been undertaken to assess the effectiveness and security of odanacatib, a phase I study to determine the dosage and a phase II study to assess the security and effectiveness. In the Phase I study a cohort of 49 women was used to assess a weekly dose. Doses of 5mg, 25mg, 50mg, and 100mg were used and 12 subjects were placed in the control cohort. A cohort of 30 women was created to enable the evaluation of the daily dosage. Doses of 0.5, 2.5, and 10mg were deployed, with six subjects placed in the control cohort. All treatments were given under fasting conditions. Odanacatib had an extended half-life of between 66 and 93 hours for all the treatments and dosages assessed. The effectiveness of both weekly and daily dosages in altering the markers was assessed. The impact was dose-dependant but not in proportion to the dosage level. Decreases in resorption markers were highest for weekly doses >50mg and daily doses ≥2.5mg. The greatest suppression was witnessed between days 3 and 5 with the weekly dose and this level remained elevated until the subsequent treatment [95].

The Phase II trial presented by Cusick et al. at the ASBMR meeting in 2009 (Denver, Co, USA), was a double-blind, randomised, controlled study lasting one year, with an expected extension period of two years. It looked at 399 postmenopausal women (postmenopausal (5yr) or bilateral oophorectomy) aged 45 to 85 years, presenting a T-score <-2 but not less than -3.5 in any one location. Subjects were assigned to five different cohorts with differing dosage levels: placebo, 3mg/week, 10mg/week, 25mg/week and 50mg/week. The variations in BMD at the lumbar spine were analysed and taken as the main outcome. In addition, variations in bone remodeling, variations in BMD in other locations and side effects were assessed in turn. The data indicated a elevation in BMD in all locations, which was related to the dose level. The more significant improvement was achieved with the highest dose. Weekly treatments of 50mg of odanacatib augmented bone mass by 5.7% in the lumbar spine, 4.1% in the total hip, 4.7% in the femoral neck, 5.2% in the trochanter and 2.9% in the distal third of the radius at the two-year point. Resorption markers dropped relative to the dose from the start of the therapy and stayed lower over the initial six-month period, at which point they increased to a similar level as those in the control group.

The data from the extension period of the phase II study to the three-year point (reported by Eisman et al. at the ASBMR meeting 2009 in Denver), looked at 169 women randomly assigned to weekly doses of odanacatib 50mg or a placebo. In the odanacatib cohort, BMD continued to rise (lumbar spine 7.5%, total hip 5.5%, femoral neck 5.5% and trochanter 7.4%). The urine NTX resorption marker was reduced by 50% versus the placebo, while the BSAP (bone specific alkaline phosphatase) formation marker remained unchanged. At the three-year point, formation markers had not only not decreased, but had in fact risen by 18% above baseline values.

6.1.4. ONO5334

ONO5334 is a new cathepsin K inhibitor. An initial trial has been carried out to assess its effectiveness and security in the treatment of postmenopausal osteoporosis. This was a year-long, randomised, double-blind, placebo and active-controlled parallel-group trial carried out across 13 locations in six European states. The study looked at 285 postmenopausal women from 55 to 75 years old with osteoporosis. Patients were randomly assigned to one of five dosage groups: placebo; 50mg twice daily, 100mg once daily, or 300mg once daily of ONO-5334; or alendronate 70mg once a week. After 12 months of monitoring all ONO-5334 doses and alendronate demonstrated a marked elevation of BMD at the lumbar spine, total hip (except the 100mg/day cohort), and femoral neck. There was little or no evidence that ONO-5334 suppressed bone-formation markers versus the alendronate, however the suppressive action on bone-resorption markers were comparable. There were no security issues of any clinic consequence. With a marked elevation in BMD, ONO-5334 also heralds a new mechanism in the treatment of osteoporosis. This new agent increases the range of treatments available both in the class of cathepsin K inhibitors as the second apparently available agent, and also across the full range of osteoporosis treatment [94].

We can conclude that Cathepsine K inhibitors are a new class of treatment that adds to the range of therapies available for the treatment and prevention of fractures, the most hazardous consequence of osteoporosis. Being able treat this condition at a variety of points along the resorption pathway is an asset and it provides clinicians with the opportunity to reduce the risk of fractures more effectively than before.

6.2. Sclerostin

Sclerostin is a protein encoded by the SOST gene [96, 97]. It is identified as an important inhibitor of osteoblast-mediated bone formation [98, 99]. Loss-of-function mutations in this gene are linked with sclerosteosis, which results in progressive bone overgrowth and elevated bone mass and BMD.

A similar condition is van Buchem disease, a less severe form of sclerostosis resulting from by a deletion downstream of this gene, and leading to reduced sclerostin expression. SOST gene knockout mice no longer produce sclerostin and have an elevated bone mass, which demonstrates the impact this protein has on bone mass and BMD levels. In addition to elevated bone mass and BMD levels resulting from sclerostin deficiency, it is notable that no fractures have been reported in patients with either sclerosteosis or van Buchem disease [99, 100].

Sclerostin binds to low-density lipoprotein receptor-related protein (LRP) 5/6 and intercepts Wnt-signaling, governing bone formation in a negative manner and preventing osteoblast differentiation, proliferation, and activity [101].

6.2.1. Anti-sclerostin monoclonal antibodies

At the present there are three separate humanized sclerostin antibodies under investigation: romosozumab (AMGEN & UCB), blozosumab (Eli Lilly) and BPS804 (Novartis). Romosozumab is a high affinity immunoglobulin G2 (IgG2) monoclonal antibody. It is produced through the humanisation of a mouse sclerostin monoclonal antibody that neutralizes sclerostin. The first-in-human single-dose trial in healthy men and postmenopausal women was carried out to assess pharmacokinetics, pharmacodynamics, tolerance and security of romosozumab doses of 0.1, 0.3, 1, 3, 5 or 10mg/kg delivered sub-cutaneously and 1 or 10mg/kg delivered intravenously. Seventy-two subjects in total took part in the trial and were subsequently monitored for a maximum of 85 days. The pharmacokinetics of this agent were not relative to the dosage levels. Dose-related rises in bone formation markers and falls in bone resorption markers were noted. A small proportion of subjects presented anti-investigational product bodies however the majority of these were non-neutralizing antibodies. The data indicated that the agent was well-tolerated [102].

In a phase II, multi-centre, multi-dose, controlled, parallel groups clinical study, 419 postmenopausal women with poor BMD were randomly assigned to the treatment to assess the effectiveness of romosozumab versus alendronate, teriparatide and a placebo, over a one year course of therapy. The main outcome was BMD change. All the dosage levels of romosozumab causes a marked elevation in the BMD at the lumbar spine, femoral neck and total hip together with a short-term rise in the bone formation markers and a durable fall in the bone resorption markers [103]. Data from the phase III studies is to be published soon.

A randomised, double-blind, controlled phase II clinical study of blosozumab in postmenopausal women with poor BMD was recently made available. Subjects were given subcutaneously administered blosozumab 180mg Q4W, 180mg Q2W, 270mg Q2W or equivalent placebo over a period of one year. In total, 120 women took part. Dosage levels across the range of blosozumab augmented lumbar spine and total hip BMD. Bone formation markers rose rapidly during the therapy while bone resorption markers fell at an early point in the therapy and continued at low level through to the end of the trial [104].

A comparable study was carried out using BPS804 with a similar cohort, however no data is yet published from this trial.

We can conclude that anti-sclerostin antibodies may be the most efficacious agent in the treatment of osteoporosis and bone defect related conditions.

7. Conclusion

Over the last decade, new drugs have come forward as potential pharmacological treatments for osteoporosis. More recent options are part of new classes of agent which present optimised modes of action, allowing practioners to replace patients' lost bone mass more quickly and efficaciously than with older treatments. Nonetheless, it is important to be aware that all drugs have their appropriate uses and also a wide range of side effects, factors which must be considered in any clinical decision-making process. Furthermore, it is vital that practitioners ensure that, as required by the majority of therapies, treatments for osteoporosis are administered alongside adjustments in a patient's lifestyle and/or calcium and vitamin D supplementation. New treatments are now coming into use that are likely to enable practitioners to opt for shorter courses of therapy which result in better outcomes for patients.

Author details

Jorge Malouf[1*], Berta Magallares[1] and Roberto Güerri[2]

*Address all correspondence to: jmalouf@santpau.cat

1 Hospital de la Santa Creu I Sant Pau, Universitat Autònoma de Barcelona, Spain

2 IMIM, Hospital del Mar, Universitat Autònoma de Barcelona, Spain

References

[1] Siris, E.S., Chen, Y.T., Abbott, T.A., Barrett-Connor, E., Miller, P.D., Wehren, L.E. and Berger, M.L., 2004. Bone mineral density thresholds for pharmacological intervention to prevent fractures. Archives of Internal Medicine, 164(10), pp. 1108-1112.

[2] Van der Wiel HE, Lips P, Nauta J, Kwakkel G, Hazenberg G, Netelenbos JC, van der Vijgh WJ. Intranasal calcitonin suppresses increased bone resorption during short-term immobilization: a double-blind study of the effects of intranasal calcitonin on biochemical parameters of bone turnover. J Bone Miner Res. 1993 Dec;8(12):1459-65.

[3] Nussbaum SR. Patrophysiology and management of severe hypercalcemia. Endocrinol Metab. Clin North Am. 1993 Jun;22(2):343-62.

[4] Lyritis GP, Trovas G. Analgesic effects of calcitonin.Bone. 2002 May;30(5 Suppl): 71S-74S. ReviewAdomaityte, J., Farooq, M. and Qayyum, R., 2008. Effect of raloxifene therapy on venous thromboembolism in postmenopausal women. A meta-analysis. Thrombosis and haemostasis, 99(2), pp. 338-342.

[5] Rossouw, J.E., Anderson, G.L., Prentice, R.L., Lacroix, A.Z., Kooperberg, C., Stefanick, M.L., Jackson, R.D., Beresford, S.A., Howard, B.V., Johnson, K.C., Kotchen, J.M., Ockene, J. and Writing Group For The Women's Health Initiative Investigators, 2002. Risks and benefits of estrogen plus progestin in healthy postmenopausal women: principal results From the Women's Health Initiative randomized controlled trial. JAMA, 288(3), pp. 321-333.

[6] Cauley, J.A., Robbins, J., Chen, Z., Cummings, S.R., Jackson, R.D., Lacroix, A.Z., Leboff, M., Lewis, C.E., Mcgowan, J., Neuner, J., Pettinger, M., Stefanick, M.L., Wactawski-Wende, J., Watts, N.B. and Women's Health Initiative Investigators, 2003. Effects

of estrogen plus progestin on risk of fracture and bone mineral density: the Women's Health Initiative randomized trial. JAMA, 290(13), pp. 1729-1738.

[7] Maclean, C., Newberry, S., Maglione, M., Mcmahon, M., Ranganath, V., Suttorp, M., Mojica, W., Timmer, M., Alexander, A., Mcnamara, M., Desai, S.B., Zhou, A., Chen, S., Carter, J., Tringale, C., Valentine, D., Johnsen, B. and Grossman, J., 2008. Systematic review: comparative effectiveness of treatments to prevent fractures in men and women with low bone density or osteoporosis. Annals of Internal Medicine, 148(3), pp. 197-213.

[8] Cauley, J.A., Black, D.M., Barrett-Connor, E., Harris, F., Shields, K., Applegate, W. and Cummings, S.R., 2001. Effects of hormone replacement therapy on clinical fractures and height loss: The Heart and Estrogen/Progestin Replacement Study (HERS). The American Journal of Medicine, 110(6), pp. 442-450.

[9] National Institute For Clinical Excellence (Nice), 2008. Systematic reviews of clinical effectiveness prepared for the guideline 'Osteoporosis: Assessment of fracture risk and the prevention of osteoporotic fractures in individuals at high risk', 2008, National Institute for Health and Clinical Excellence.

[10] Wimalawansa, S.J., 1998. A four-year randomized controlled trial of hormone replacement and bisphosphonate, alone or in combination, in women with postmenopausal osteoporosis. The American Journal of Medicine, 104(3), pp. 219-226.

[11] Mosekilde, L., Beck-Nielsen, H., Sorensen, O.H., Nielsen, S.P., Charles, P., Vestergaard, P., Hermann, A.P., Gram, J., Hansen, T.B., Abrahamsen, B., Ebbesen, E.N., Stilgren, L., Jensen, L.B., Brot, C., Hansen, B., Tofteng, C.L., Eiken, P. and Kolthoff, N., 2000. Hormonal replacement therapy reduces forearm fracture incidence in recent postmenopausal women - results of the Danish Osteoporosis Prevention Study. Maturitas, 36(3), pp. 181-193.

[12] Anderson, D.M., Maraskovsky, E., Billingsley, W.L., Dougall, W.C., Tometsko, M.E., Roux, E.R., Teepe, M.C., Dubose, R.F., Cosman, D. and Galibert, L., 1997. A homologue of the TNF receptor and its ligand enhance T-cell growth and dendritic-cell function. Nature, 390(6656), pp. 175-179.

[13] Lufkin, E.G., Wahner, H.W., O'fallon, W.M., Hodgson, S.F., Kotowicz, M.A., Lane, A.W., Judd, H.L., Caplan, R.H. and Riggs, B.L., 1992. Treatment of postmenopausal osteoporosis with transdermal estrogen. Annals of Internal Medicine, 117(1), pp. 1-9.

[14] Anderson, G.L., Judd, H.L., Kaunitz, A.M., Barad, D.H., Beresford, S.A., Pettinger, M., Liu, J., Mcneeley, S.G., Lopez, A.M. and Women's Health Initiative Investigators, 2003. Effects of estrogen plus progestin on gynecologic cancers and associated diagnostic procedures: the Women's Health Initiative randomized trial. JAMA, 290(13), pp. 1739-1748.

[15] Herrington, D.M., Reboussin, D.M., Brosnihan, K.B., Sharp, P.C., Shumaker, S.A., Snyder, T.E., Furberg, C.D., Kowalchuk, G.J., Stuckey, T.D., Rogers, W.J., Givens,

D.H. and Waters, D., 2000. Effects of estrogen replacement on the progression of coronary-artery atherosclerosis. The New England journal of medicine, 343(8), pp. 522-529.

[16] Ravn, P., Bidstrup, M., Wasnich, R.D., Davis, J.W., Mcclung, M.R., Balske, A., Coupland, C., Sahota, O., Kaur, A., Daley, M. and Cizza, G., 1999. Alendronate and estrogen-progestin in the long-term prevention of bone loss: four-year results from the early postmenopausal intervention cohort study. A randomized, controlled trial. Annals of Internal Medicine, 131(12), pp. 935-942.

[17] Cherry, N., Gilmour, K., Hannaford, P., Heagerty, A., Khan, M.A., Kitchener, H., Mcnamee, R., Elstein, M., Kay, C., Seif, M., Buckley, H. and Esprit Team, 2002. Oestrogen therapy for prevention of reinfarction in postmenopausal women: a randomised placebo controlled trial. Lancet, 360(9350), pp. 2001-2008.

[18] Hulley, S., Grady, D., Bush, T., Furberg, C., Herrington, D., Riggs, B. and Vittinghoff, E.,1998. Randomized trial of estrogen plus progestin for secondary prevention of coronary heart disease in postmenopausal women. Heart and Estrogen/progestin Replacement Study (HERS) Research Group. JAMA, 280(7), pp. 605-613.

[19] Stampfer, M.J., Colditz, G.A., Willett, W.C., Manson, J.E., Rosner, B., Speizer, F.E. and Hennekens, C.H., 1991. Postmenopausal estrogen therapy and cardiovascular disease. Ten-year follow-up from the nurses' health study. The New England journal of medicine, 325(11), pp. 756-762.

[20] Grady, D., Gebretsadik, T., Kerlikowske, K., Ernster, V. and Petitti, D., 1995. Hormone replacement therapy and endometrial cancer risk: a meta-analysis. Obstetrics and gynecology, 85(2), pp. 304-313.

[21] Barrett-Connor, E., 1992. Risks and benefits of replacement estrogen. Annual Review of Medicine, 43, pp. 239-251.

[22] Humphrey, L.L., Chan, B.K. and Sox, H.C., 2002. Postmenopausal hormone replacement therapy and the primary prevention of cardiovascular disease. Annals of Internal Medicine, 137(4), pp. 273-284.

[23] Viscoli, C.M., Brass, L.M., Kernan, W.N., Sarrel, P.M., Suissa, S. and Horwitz, R.I., 2001. A clinical trial of estrogen-replacement therapy after ischemic stroke. The New England journal of medicine, 345(17), pp. 1243-1249.

[24] Miller, J., Chan, B.K. and Nelson, H.D., 2002. Postmenopausal estrogen replacement and risk for venous thromboembolism: a systematic review and meta-analysis for the U.S. Preventive Services Task Force. Annals of Internal Medicine, 136(9), pp. 680-690.

[25] Lethaby, A., Suckling, J., Barlow, D., Farquhar, C.M., Jepson, R.G. and Roberts, H., 2004. Hormone replacement therapy in postmenopausal women: endometrial hyperplasia and irregular bleeding. Cochrane database of systematic reviews (Online), (3) (3), pp. CD000402.

[26] Nelson, H.D., 2004. Commonly used types of postmenopausal estrogen for treatment of hot flashes: scientific review. JAMA : the journal of the American Medical Association, 291(13), pp. 1610-1620.

[27] Garg, P.P., Kerlikowske, K., Subak, L. and Grady, D., 1998. Hormone Replacement Therapy and the Risk of Epithelial Ovarian Carcinoma: A Meta-Analysis. Obstetrics & Gynecology, 92(3),.

[28] Negri, E., Tzonou, A., Beral, V., Lagiou, P., Trichopoulos, D., Parazzini, F., Franceschi, S., Booth, M. and La Vecchia, C., 1999. Hormonal therapy for menopause and ovarian cancer in a collaborative re-analysis of European studies. International journal of cancer.Journal international du cancer, 80(6), pp. 848-851.

[29] Lacey, J.V.,Jr, Mink, P.J., Lubin, J.H., Sherman, M.E., Troisi, R., Hartge, P., Schatzkin, A. and Schairer, C., 2002. Menopausal hormone replacement therapy and risk of ovarian cancer. JAMA, 288(3), pp. 334-341.

[30] Rodriguez, C., Patel, A.V., Calle, E.E., Jacob, E.J. and Thun, M.J., 2001. Estrogen replacement therapy and ovarian cancer mortality in a large prospective study of US women. JAMA : the journal of the American Medical Association, 285(11), pp. 1460-1465.

[31] Cranney, A., Tugwell, P., Zytaruk, N., Robinson, V., Weaver, B., Adachi, J., Wells, G., Shea, B., Guyatt, G. And Osteoporosis Methodology Group and the Osteoporosis Research Advisory Group, 2002. Meta-analyses of therapies for postmenopausal osteoporosis. IV. Meta-analysis of raloxifene for the prevention and treatment of postmenopausal osteoporosis. Endocrine reviews, 23(4), pp. 524-528.

[32] Delmas, P.D., Bjarnason, N.H., Mitlak, B.H., Ravoux, A.C., Shah, A.S., Huster, W.J., Draper, M. and Christiansen, C., 1997. Effects of raloxifene on bone mineral density, serum cholesterol concentrations, and uterine endometrium in postmenopausal women. The New England journal of medicine, 337(23), pp. 1641-1647.

[33] Burshell, A.L., Song, J., Dowsett, S.A., Mershon, J.L., Delmas, P.D., Secrest, R.J. and Cauley, J.A., 2008. Relationship between bone mass, invasive breast cancer incidence and raloxifene therapy in postmenopausal women with low bone mass or osteoporosis. Current medical research and opinion, 24(3), pp. 807-813.

[34] Martino, S., Disch, D., Dowsett, S.A., Keech, C.A. and Mershon, J.L., 2005. Safety assessment of raloxifene over eight years in a clinical trial setting. Current medical research and opinion, 21(9), pp. 1441-1452.

[35] Adomaityte, J., Farooq, M. and Qayyum, R., 2008. Effect of raloxifene therapy on venous thromboembolism in postmenopausal women. A meta-analysis. Thrombosis and haemostasis, 99(2), pp. 338-342.

[36] Collins, P., Mosca, L., Geiger, M.J., Grady, D., Kornitzer, M., Amewou-Atisso, M.G., Effron, M.B., Dowsett, S.A., Barrett-Connor, E. and Wenger, N.K., 2009. Effects of the selective estrogen receptor modulator raloxifene on coronary outcomes in the Raloxi-

fene Use for The Heart trial: results of subgroup analyses by age and other factors. Circulation, 119(7), pp. 922-930.

[37] Vogel, V.G., Costantino, J.P., Wickerham, D.L., Cronin, W.M., Cecchini, R.S., Atkins, J.N., Bevers, T.B., Fehrenbacher, L., Pajon, E.R.,Jr, Wade, J.L.,3rd, Robidoux, A., Margolese, R.G., James, J., Lippman, S.M., Runowicz, C.D., Ganz, P.A., Reis, S.E., Mccaskill-Stevens, W., Ford, L.G., Jordan, V.C., Wolmark, N. and National Surgical Adjuvant Breast And Bowel Project (Nsabp), 2006. Effects of tamoxifen vs raloxifene on the risk of developing invasive breast cancer and other disease outcomes: the NSABP Study of Tamoxifen and Raloxifene (STAR) P-2 trial. JAMA, 295(23), pp. 2727-2741.

[38] Gruber, C. and Gruber, D., 2004. Bazedoxifene (Wyeth). Current opinion in investigational drugs (London, England : 2000), 5(10), pp. 1086-1093.

[39] Pinkerton, J.V., Archer, D.F., Utian, W.H., Menegoci, J.C., Levine, A.B., Chines, A.A. and Constantine, G.D., 2009. Bazedoxifene effects on the reproductive tract in postmenopausal women at risk for osteoporosis. Menopause (New York, N.Y.), 16(6), pp. 1102-1108.

[40] Miller, P.D., Chines, A.A., Christiansen, C., Hoeck, H.C., Kendler, D.L., Lewiecki, E.M., Woodson, G., Levine, A.B., Constantine, G. and Delmas, P.D., 2008. Effects of bazedoxifene on BMD and bone turnover in postmenopausal women: 2-yr results of a randomized, double-blind, placebo-, and active-controlled study. Journal of bone and mineral research, 23(4), pp. 525-535.

[41] Silverman, S.L., Christiansen, C., Genant, H.K., Vukicevic, S., Zanchetta, J.R., De Villiers, T.J., Constantine, G.D. and Chines, A.A., 2008. Efficacy of bazedoxifene in reducing new vertebral fracture risk in postmenopausal women with osteoporosis: results from a 3-year, randomized, placebo-, and active-controlled clinical trial. Journal of bone and mineral research, 23(12), pp. 1923-1934.

[42] Mitwally, M.F., 2008. Bazedoxifene: a selective estrogen-receptor modulator. Women's health (London, England), 4(4), pp. 319-326.

[43] Clarke, B.L. and Khosla, S., 2009. New selective estrogen and androgen receptor modulators. Current opinion in rheumatology, 21(4), pp. 374-379.

[44] Harris ST. Bisphosphonates for the treatment of postmenopausal osteoporosis: clinical studies of etidronate and alendronate. Osteoporos Int. 2001 Dec;12 Suppl 3:S11-6.

[45] Guañabens N, Farrerons J, Perez-Edo L, Monegal A, Renau A, Carbonell J, Roca M, Torra M, Pavesi M. Cyclical etidronate versus sodium fluoride in established postmenopausal osteoporosis: a randomized 3 year trial. Bone. 2000 Jul;27(1):123-8

[46] McCloskey, E., Selby, P., Davies, M., Robinson, J., Francis, R.M., Adams, J., Kayan, K., Beneton, M., Jalava, T., Pylkkanen, L., Kenraali, J., Aropuu, S. and Kanis, J.A., 2004. Clodronate reduces vertebral fracture risk in women with postmenopausal or

http://dx.doi.org/10.5772/59469

secondary osteoporosis: results of a double-blind, placebo-controlled 3-year study. Journal of bone and mineral research, 19(5), pp. 728-736.

[47] Black, D.M., Cummings, S.R., Karpf, D.B., Cauley, J.A., Thompson, D.E., Nevitt, M.C., Bauer, D.C., Genant, H.K., Haskell, W.L., Marcus, R., Ott, S.M., Torner, J.C., Quandt, S.A., Reiss, T.F. and Ensrud, K.E., 1996. Randomised trial of effect of alendronate on risk of fracture in women with existing vertebral fractures. Fracture Intervention Trial Research Group. Lancet, 348(9041), Pp. 1535-1541.

[48] Levis, S., Quandt, S.A., Thompson, D., Scott, J., Schneider, D.L., Ross, P.D., Black, D., Suryawanshi, S., Hochberg, M., Yates, J. and Fit Research Group, 2002. Alendronate reduces the risk of multiple symptomatic fractures: results from the fracture intervention trial. Journal of the American Geriatrics Society, 50(3), pp. 409-415.

[49] Bauer, D.C., Black, D.M., Garnero, P., Hochberg, M., Ott, S., Orloff, J., Thompson, D.E., Ewing, S.K., Delmas, P.D. and Fracture Intervention Trial Study Group, 2004. Change in bone turnover and hip, non-spine, and vertebral fracture in alendronate-treated women: the fracture intervention trial. Journal of bone and mineral research, 19(8), pp. 1250-1258.

[50] Chapurlat, R.D., Palermo, L., Ramsay, P. and Cummings, S.R., 2005. Risk of fracture among women who lose bone density during treatment with alendronate. The Fracture Intervention Trial. Osteoporosis international, 16(7), pp. 842-848.

[51] Quandt, S.A., Thompson, D.E., Schneider, D.L., Nevitt, M.C., Black, D.M. and Fracture Intervention Trial Research Group, 2005. Effect of alendronate on vertebral fracture risk in women with bone mineral density T scores of-1.6 to -2.5 at the femoral neck: the Fracture Intervention Trial. Mayo Clinic proceedings.Mayo Clinic, 80(3), pp. 343-349.

[52] McClung, M.R., Geusens, P., Miller, P.D., Zippel, H., Bensen, W.G., Roux, C., Adami, S., Fogelman, I., Diamond, T., Eastell, R., Meunier, P.J., Reginster, J.Y. and Hip Intervention Program Study Group, 2001. Effect of risedronate on the risk of hip fracture in elderly women. Hip Intervention Program Study Group. The New England journal of medicine, 344(5), pp. 333-340.

[53] Reginster, J., Minne, H.W., Sorensen, O.H., Hooper, M., Roux, C., Brandi, M.L., Lund, B., Ethgen, D., Pack, S., Roumagnac, I. and Eastell, R., 2000. Randomized trial of the effects of risedronate on vertebral fractures in women with established postmenopausal osteoporosis. Vertebral Efficacy with Risedronate Therapy (VERT) Study Group. Osteoporosis international, 11(1), pp. 83-91.

[54] Chesnut, C.H., 2006. Treating osteoporosis with bisphosphonates and addressing adherence: a review of oral ibandronate. Drugs, 66(10), pp. 1351-1359

[55] Delmas, P.D., Recker, R.R., Chesnut, C.H.,3rd, Skag, A., Stakkestad, J.A., Emkey, R., Gilbride, J., Schimmer, R.C. and Christiansen, C., 2004. Daily and intermittent oral ibandronate normalize bone turnover and provide significant reduction in vertebral

fracture risk: results from the BONE study. Osteoporosis international, 15(10), pp. 792-798.

[56] Lyles, K.W., Colon-Emeric, C.S., Magaziner, J.S., Adachi, J.D., Pieper, C.F., Mautalen, C., Hyldstrup, L., Recknor, C., Nordsletten, L., Moore, K.A., Lavecchia, C., Zhang, J., Mesenbrink, P., Hodgson, P.K., Abrams, K., Orloff, J.J., Horowitz, Z., Eriksen, E.F., Boonen, S. and Horizon Recurrent Fracture Trial, 2007. Zoledronic acid and clinical fractures and mortality after hip fracture. The New England journal of medicine, 357(18), pp. 1799-1809.

[57] Black, D.M., Delmas, P.D., Eastell, R., Reid, I.R., Boonen, S., Cauley, J.A., Cosman, F., Lakatos, P., Leung, P.C., Man, Z., Mautalen, C., Mesenbrink, P., Hu, H., Caminis, J., Tong, K., Rosario-Jansen, T., Krasnow, J., Hue, T.F., Sellmeyer, D., Eriksen, E.F., Cummings, S.R. and Horizon Pivotal Fracture Trial, 2007. Once-yearly zoledronic acid for treatment of postmenopausal osteoporosis. The New England journal of medicine, 356(18), pp. 1809-1822.

[58] Marx, R.E., 2003. Pamidronate (Aredia) and zoledronate (Zometa) induced avascular necrosis of the jaws: a growing epidemic. Journal of oral and maxillofacial surgery, 61(9), pp. 1115-1117.

[59] Schilcher J, Michaëlsson K, Aspenberg P. Bisphosphonate use and atypical fractures of the femoral shaft. N Engl J Med. 2011 May 5;364(18):1728-37.

[60] Bone, H.G., Bolognese, M.A., Yuen, C.K., Kendler, D.L., Wang, H., Liu, Y. and San Martin, J., 2008. Effects of denosumab on bone mineral density and bone turnover in postmenopausal women. The Journal of clinical endocrinology and metabolism, 93(6), pp. 2149-2157.

[61] Brown, J.P., Prince, R.L., Deal, C., Recker, R.R., Kiel, D.P., De Gregorio, L.H., Hadji, P., Hofbauer, L.C., Alvaro-Gracia, J.M., Wang, H., Austin, M., Wagman, R.B., Newmark, R., Libanati, C., San Martin, J. and Bone, H.G., 2009. Comparison of the Effect of Denosumab and Alendronate on Bone Mineral Density and Biochemical Markers of Bone Turnover in Postmenopausal Women With Low Bone Mass: A Randomized, Blinded, Phase 3 Trial. Journal of bone and mineral research, pp. 1-34.

[62] Kendler, D.L., Roux, C., Benhamou, C.L., Brown, J.P., Lillestol, M., Siddhanti, S., Man, H.S., San Martin, J. and Bone, H.G., 2010. Effects of denosumab on bone mineral density and bone turnover in postmenopausal women transitioning from alendronate therapy. Journal of bone and mineral research, 25(1), pp. 72-81.

[63] Scott LJ. Denosumab: a review of its use in postmenopausal women with osteoporosis. Drugs Aging. 2014 Jul;31(7):555-76.

[64] Pandey, J. and Pandey, U., 2011. Fluoride Contamination and Fluorosis in Rural Community in the Vicinity of a Phosphate Fertilizer Factory in India. Bulletin of environmental contamination and toxicology..

[65] Turner, C.H., 1996. *Fluoride and the FDA: a curious case.* Journal of bone and mineral research, *(9), pp. 1369-1371.*

[66] Farrerons, J., Rodriguez De La Serna, A., Guanabens, N., Armadans, L., Lopez-Navidad, A., Yoldi, B., Renau, A. and Vaque, J., 1997. Sodium fluoride treatment is a major protector against vertebral and nonvertebral fractures when compared with other common treatments of osteoporosis: a longitudinal, observational study. Calcified tissue international, 60(3), pp. 250-254.

[67] Haguenauer, D., Welch, V., Shea, B., Tugwell, P., Adachi, J.D. and Wells, G., 2000a. Fluoride for the treatment of postmenopausal osteoporotic fractures: a meta-analysis. Osteoporosis 11(9), pp. 727-738.

[68] Haguenauer, D., Welch, V., Shea, B., Tugwell, P. and Wells, G., 2000b. Fluoride for treating postmenopausal osteoporosis. Cochrane database of systematic reviews.

[69] Dempster, D.W., Cosman, F., Kurland, E.S., Zhou, H., Nieves, J., Woelfert, L., Shane, E., Plavetic, K., Muller, R., Bilezikian, J. and Lindsay, R., 2001. Effects of daily treatment with parathyroid hormone on bone microarchitecture and turnover in patients with osteoporosis: a paired biopsy study. Journal of bone and mineral research: the official journal of the American Society for Bone and Mineral Research, 16(10), pp. 1846-1853.

[70] Keaveny, T.M., Donley, D.W., Hoffmann, P.F., Mitlak, B.H., Glass, E.V. and San Martin, J.A., 2007. Effects of teriparatide and alendronate on vertebral strength as assessed by finite element modeling of QCT scans in women with osteoporosis. Journal of bone and mineral research, 22(1), pp. 149-157.

[71] Hodsman, A.B., Bauer, D.C., Dempster, D.W., Dian, L., Hanley, D.A., Harris, S.T., Kendler, D.L., Mcclung, M.R., Miller, P.D., Olszynski, W.P., Orwoll, E. and Yuen, C.K., 2005. Parathyroid hormone and teriparatide for the treatment of osteoporosis: a review of the evidence and suggested guidelines for its use. Endocrine reviews, 26(5), pp. 688-703.

[72] Neer, R.M., Arnaud, C.D., Zanchetta, J.R., Prince, R., Gaich, G.A., Reginster, J.Y., Hodsman, A.B., Eriksen, E.F., Ish-Shalom, S., Genant, H.K., Wang, O. and Mitlak, B.H., 2001. Effect of parathyroid hormone (1-34) on fractures and bone mineral density in postmenopausal women with osteoporosis. The New England journal of medicine, 344(19), pp. 1434-1441.

[73] Vahle, J.L., Long, G.G., Sandusky, G., Westmore, M., Ma, Y.L. and Sato, M., 2004. Bone neoplasms in F344 rats given teriparatide [rhPTH(1-34)] are dependent on duration of treatment and dose. Toxicologic pathology, 32(4), pp. 426-438.

[74] Lindsay, R., Scheele, W.H., Neer, R., Pohl, G., Adami, S., Mautalen, C., Reginster, J.Y., Stepan, J.J., Myers, S.L. and Mitlak, B.H., 2004. Sustained vertebral fracture risk reduction after withdrawal of teriparatide in postmenopausal women with osteoporosis. Archives of Internal Medicine, 164(18), pp. 2024-2030.

[75] Finkelstein, J.S., Hayes, A., Hunzelman, J.L., Wyland, J.J., Lee, H. and Neer, R.M., 2003. The effects of parathyroid hormone, alendronate, or both in men with osteoporosis. The New England journal of medicine, 349(13), pp. 1216-1226.

[76] Jn T, Av U, Sm BB, Rm N, Y Z, N D, H L, Ml B, Bz L. Comparative Effects of Teriparatide, Denosumab, and Combination Therapy on Peripheral Compartmental Bone Density, Microarchitecture, and Estimated Strength: the DATA-HRpQCT Study. J Bone Miner Res. 2014 Jul 17.

[77] Obermayer-Pietsch, B.M., Marin, F., Mccloskey, E.V., Hadji, P., Farrerons, J., Boonen, S., Audran, M., Barker, C., Anastasilakis, A.D., Fraser, W.D., Nickelsen, T. and Eurofors Investigators, 2008. Effects of two years of daily teriparatide treatment on BMD in postmenopausal women with severe osteoporosis with and without prior antiresorptive treatment. Journal of bone and mineral research, 23(10), pp. 1591-1600.

[78] Ettinger, B., San Martin, J., Crans, G. and Pavo, I., 2004. Differential effects of teriparatide on BMD after treatment with raloxifene or alendronate. Journal of bone and mineral research, 19(5), pp. 745-751.

[79] Saag, K.G., Zanchetta, J.R., Devogelaer, J.P., Adler, R.A., Eastell, R., See, K., Krege, J.H., Krohn, K. and Warner, M.R., 2009. Effects of teriparatide versus alendronate for treating glucocorticoid-induced osteoporosis: thirty-six-month results of a randomized, double-blind, controlled trial. Arthritis and Rheumatism, 60(11), pp. 3346-3355.

[80] Orwoll, E.S., Scheele, W.H., Paul, S., Adami, S., Syversen, U., Diez-Perez, A., Kaufman, J.M., Clancy, A.D. and Gaich, G.A., 2003. The effect of teriparatide [human parathyroid hormone (1-34)] therapy on bone density in men with osteoporosis. Journal of bone and mineral research, 18(1), pp. 9-17.

[81] Rosen, C.J. and Bilezikian, J.P., 2001. Clinical review 123: Anabolic therapy for osteoporosis. The Journal of clinical endocrinology and metabolism, 86(3), pp. 957-964.

[82] Giammarile, F., Mognetti, T., Blondet, C., Desuzinges, C. and Chauvot, P., 1999. Bone pain palliation with 85Sr therapy. Journal of nuclear medicine, 40(4), pp. 585-590.

[83] Saarto, T., Janes, R., Tenhunen, M. and Kouri, M., 2002. Palliative radiotherapy in the treatment of skeletal metastases. European journal of pain (London, England), 6(5), pp. 323-330.

[84] Bonnelye, E., Chabadel, A., Saltel, F. and Jurdic, P., 2008. Dual effect of strontium ranelate: stimulation of osteoblast differentiation and inhibition of osteoclast formation and resorption in vitro. Bone, 42(1), pp. 129-138.

[85] Close, P., Neuprez, A. and Reginster, J.Y., 2006. Developments in the pharmacotherapeutic management of osteoporosis. Expert Opin Pharmacother, 7(12), pp. 1603-15.

[86] Chapurlat, R. and Delmas, P.D., 2004. *New treatments in osteoporosis.* La Revue de medecine interne / fondee par la Societe nationale francaise de medecine interne,, *pp. S573-9.*

[87] Blake, G.M. and Fogelman, I., 2006. Theoretical model for the interpretation of BMD scans in patients stopping strontium ranelate treatment. Journal of bone and mineral research, 21(9), pp. 1417-1424.

[88] Reginster, J.Y., Seeman, E., De Vernejoul, M.C., Adami, S., Compston, J., Phenekos, C., Devogelaer, J.P., Curiel, M.D., Sawicki, A., Goemaere, S., Sorensen, O.H., Felsenberg, D. and Meunier, P.J., 2005. Strontium ranelate reduces the risk of nonvertebral fractures in postmenopausal women with osteoporosis: Treatment of Peripheral Osteoporosis (TROPOS) study. J Clin Endocrinol Metab, 90(5), pp. 2816-22.

[89] Reginster, J.Y., Felsenberg, D., Boonen, S., Diez-Perez, A., Rizzoli, R., Brandi, M.L., Spector, T.D., Brixen, K., Goemaere, S., Cormier, C., Balogh, A., Delmas, P.D. and Meunier, P.J., 2008. Effects of long-term strontium ranelate treatment on the risk of nonvertebral and vertebral fractures in postmenopausal osteoporosis: Results of a five-year, randomized, placebo-controlled trial. Arthritis and Rheumatism, 58(6), pp. 1687-1695.

[90] Moro-Alvarez, M.J. and Diaz-Curiel, M., 2007. Pharmacological treatment of osteoporosis for people over 70. Aging clinical and experimental research, 19(3), pp. 246-254.

[91] Bromme, D. and Lecaille, F., 2009. Cathepsin K inhibitors for osteoporosis and potential off-target effects. Expert opinion on investigational drugs, 18(5), pp. 585-600.

[92] Jerome C, Missbach M, Gamse R. Balicatib, a cathepsin K inhibitor, stimulates periosteal bone formation in monkeys. Osteoporos Int. 2011 Dec;22(12):3001-11.

[93] Stroup GB, Kumar S, Jerome CP. Treatment with a potent cathepsin K inhibitor preserves cortical and trabecular bone mass in ovariectomized monkeys. Calcif Tissue Int. 2009 Oct;85(4):344-55.

[94] Eastell, R., Nagase, S., Ohyama, M., Small, M., Sawyer, J., Boonen, S., Spector, T., Kuwayama, T. and Deacon, S., 2011. Safety and efficacy of the cathepsin K inhibitor ONO-5334 in postmenopausal osteoporosis: the OCEAN study. Journal of bone and mineral research, 26(6), pp. 1303-1312.

[95] Stoch, S.A., Zajic, S., Stone, J., Miller, D.L., Van Dyck, K., Gutierrez, M.J., De Decker, M., Liu, L., Liu, Q., Scott, B.B., Panebianco, D., Jin, B., Duong, L.T., Gottesdiener, K. and Wagner, J.A., 2009. Effect of the cathepsin K inhibitor odanacatib on bone resorption biomarkers in healthy postmenopausal women: two double-blind, randomized, placebo-controlled phase I studies. Clinical pharmacology and therapeutics, 86(2), pp. 175-182.

[96] Balemans, W., Ebeling, M., Patel, N., Van Hul, E., Olson, P., Dioszegi, M., Lacza, C., Wuyts, W., Van Den Ende, J., Willems, P., Paes-Alves, A.F., Hill, S., Bueno, M., Ramos, F.J., Tacconi, P., Dikkers, F.G., Stratakis, C., Lindpaintner, K., Vickery, B., Foernzler, D. and Van Hul, W., 2001. Increased bone density in sclerosteosis is due to the deficiency of a novel secreted protein (SOST). Human molecular genetics, 10(5), pp. 46 537-543.

[97] Brunkow, M.E., Gardner, J.C., Van Ness, J., Paeper, B.W., Kovacevich, B.R., Proll, S., Skonier, J.E., Zhao, L., Sabo, P.J., Fu, Y., Alisch, R.S., Gillett, L., Colbert, T., Tacconi, P., Galas, D., Hamersma, H., Beighton, P. and Mulligan, J., 2001. Bone dysplasia sclerosteosis results from loss of the SOST gene product, a novel cystine knot containing protein. American Journal of Human Genetics, 68(3), pp. 577-589.

[98] Poole, K.E., Van Bezooijen, R.L., Loveridge, N., Hamersma, H., Papapoulos, S.E., Lowik, C.W. and Reeve, J., 2005. Sclerostin is a delayed secreted product of osteocytes that inhibits bone formation. The FASEB journal, 19(13), pp. 1842-1844.

[99] Wergedal, J.E., Veskovic, K., Hellan, M., Nyght, C., Balemans, W., Libanati, C., Vanhoenacker, F.M., Tan, J., Baylink, D.J. And Van Hul, W., 2003. Patients with Van Buchem disease, an osteosclerotic genetic disease, have elevated bone formation markers, higher bone density, and greater derived polar moment of inertia than normal. The Journal of clinical endocrinology and metabolism, 88(12), pp. 5778-5783.

[100] Hamersma, H., Gardner, J. and Beighton, P., 2003. The natural history of sclerosteosis. Clinical genetics, 63(3), pp. 192-197.

[101] Baron, R. and Rawadi, G., 2007. Targeting the Wnt/beta-catenin pathway to regulate bone formation in the adult skeleton. Endocrinology, 148(6), pp. 2635-2643.

[102] Padhi, D., Jang, G., Stouch, B., Fang, L. and Posvar, E., 2011. Single-dose, placebo-controlled, randomized study of AMG 785, a sclerostin monoclonal antibody. Journal of bone and mineral research, 26(1), pp. 19-26.

[103] McClung MR, Grauer A. Romosozumab in postmenopausal women with osteopenia. N Engl J Med. 2014 Apr 24;370(17):1664-5.

[104] Recker R, Benson C, Matsumoto T, Bolognese M, Robins D, Alam J, Chiang AY, Hu L, Krege JH, Sowa H, Mitlak B, Myers S. A randomized, double-blind phase 2 clinical trial of blosozumab, a sclerostin antibody, in postmenopausal women with low bone mineral density. J Bone Miner Res. 2014 Sep 5.

Chapter 7

Management of Osteoporosis in Chronic Kidney Diseases

Vinita Mishra

Additional information is available at the end of the chapter

http://dx.doi.org/10.5772/59607

1. Introduction

1.1. Chronic kidney disease (CKD)

Chronic kidney disease (CKD) is an international public health problem affecting 5–10% of the world population, as it is responsible for high morbidity and mortality particularly affecting population over 60 years of age. [1]. CKD is defined as abnormal renal function or structure [1].

GFR category	GFR (ml/min/1.73 m ^{2})	Terms
G1	>90	Normal or high
G2	60–89	Mildly decreased*
G3a	45–59	Mildly to moderately decreased
G3b	30–44	Moderately to severely decreased
G4	15–29	Severely decreased
G5	<15	Kidney failure

* Relative to young adult level

Abbreviations: CKD, chronic kidney disease; GFR, glomerular filtration rate

Reprinted with permission from Kidney Disease: Improving Global Outcomes (KDIGO) CKD Work Group (2013) KDIGO 2012 clinical practice guideline for the evaluation and management of chronic kidney disease. Kidney International (Suppl. 3): 1–150

Table 1. Stages in CKD

As classified by National Kidney Foundation [1] and Kidney disease improving global outcome (KDIGO) [2] CKD has 5 stages based on e GFR (estimated glomerular filtration rate) (Table 1) and markers of kidney damage. CKD is diagnosed when e GFR is consistently <60ml/min/1.73^2 on at least two separate occasion separated by a period of more than 3 months. Stage 3 is further sub classified into 3a (45 to 59ml/min) and 3b (30 to 44ml/min) and includes albuminuria in the classification. eGFR ≥30-60ml/min/1.73^2 or stage 3 is referred as "early CKD" and eGFR <30 or stage 4-5 is referred as "late CKD". Stage 5 or e GFR <15 is also referred as end stage renal disease (ESRD).

1.2. Bone mineral disruption in CKD

As kidney function declines, there is a progressive deterioration in mineral homeostasis, with a disruption of normal serum concentrations of calcium and phosphorus. The disturbance in mineral homeostasis is due to changes in circulating levels of hormones such as parathyroid hormone (PTH), 25-hydroxyvitamin D [25 (OH) D), 1,25-dihydroxyvitamin D [1,25 (OH) D)or calcitriol and fibroblast growth factor (FGF-23] [3].

Beginning in CKD stage 3 or early CKD, the ability of the kidney to appropriately excrete a phosphate load is diminished. However, serum calcium and phosphorous levels remain within the reference range with PTH either within the reference range or slightly elevated. Rise in FGF-23appears much earlier than changes in serum phosphate or PTH [4,5]. FGF-23 is produced by osteocytes and osteoblasts. It has phosphaturic action where by it reduces the renal tubular reabsorption of phosphate by reducing the expression of sodium phosphate cotransporters in renal tubule through Klotho-FGF receptor. Therefore, FGF-23 production is stimulated by impaired renal excretion of phosphate and elevated 1,25 (OH)D.FGF-23 indirectly stimulates PTH secretion by decreasing the synthesis of 1,25 (OH)D. Studies have shown the effect of this raised FGF-23 on mortality in dialysis patients [6].

As CKD progresses further, hyperphosphatemia stimulates the secretion of PTH, leading to secondary hyperparathyroidism. Additionally, hyperphosphatemia itself has direct posttranslational effect on PTH synthesis [7]. Further deterioration in kidney function results in impaired conversion of 25 (OH) D) to 1,25 (OH) D, reducing 1,25 (OH)Dsynthesis. This reducesintestinal calcium absorption and ensuing hypocalcaemia further stimulates PTH secretion aggravating secondary hyperparathyroidism. FGF-23 also down regulates the synthesis of 1,25 (OH)D through 1-alfa hydroxylase, which exacerbates the secondary hyperparathyroidism. In addition, there is evidence at the tissue level of a down regulation of vitamin D receptor and of resistance to the actions of PTH. Due to target tissue resistance to PTH action, kidney fails to respond adequately toPTH, aggravating secondary hyperparathyroidism.

Thus there is continuous secretion of PTH due to hyperphosphatemia, hypocalcaemia, reduced synthesis of 1,25 (OH)D resulting in parathyroid hyperplasia [8]. This is commonly seen in late CKD, which presents with mineral and hormonal disturbances such as hypocalcaemia, hyperphosphatemia, raised PTH, raised FGF-23 and low vitamin D status.

The disruption in mineral and endocrine functions in CKD has significant effect on bone remodeling as secondary hyperparathyroidism stimulates the bone resorption. Vitamin D deficiency disrupts mineralization of bone leading to overall deterioration in bone quality.Hence a wide spectrum of bone metabolic disorders is seen in patients with CKD stage 3-5 and those on dialysis (stage 5D). This mineral and hormonal disruption in CKD alters the bone morphology and constitutes renal osteodystrophy of CKD.PTH and vitamin D are the major hormones, which, are involved in renal osteodystrophy. Besides this recent studies have shown that FGF-23 also contributes to vitamin D deficiency [10].More recently, there has been an increasing concern for extra skeletal calcification that may result from the deranged mineral and bone metabolism of CKD. Extra skeletal calcification or vascular calcifications is major risk for cardiovascular disease in CKD patients contributing to high morbidity and mortality in this sub population group.

1.3. Bone metabolic disorders in CKD

CKD can present with wide spectrum of bone metabolic disorders, includingrenal osteodystrophy and osteoporosis. The manifestation of bone metabolic disorders is influenced by the severity of CKD. Osteoporosis is predominant in early CKD where it is potentiated by risk factors such as ageing, gender (post menopausal women), poor calcium and vitamin D intake, premature menopause, medications and chronic inflammatory disorders. These risk factors reduces the bone mass and results in osteoporosis. Renal osteodystrophy is predominant in late CKD where impaired bone and mineral homeostasis associated with hormonal disturbances affects the bone quality and mineralization. Both types of bone metabolic disorders increase the risk of bone fragility fractures thereby contributing to high morbidity and mortality in CKD patients.

1.3.1. Osteoporosis

Osteoporosis, which is characterized by low bone mass, is traditionally diagnosed as low bone mineral density (BMD). Osteoporosis as defined by WHO is the measurement of bone density at lumbar spine or hip which is equal to or less than 2.5 standard below the bone density of young adult reference population.DEXA or dual energy X ray absorptiometry is recommended as a diagnostic tool for measuring BMD. Osteoporosis is more common in postmenopausal women particularly Caucasian women [11].Pathologically, osteoporosis is associated with high bone turnover due to increased osteoclastic activity, increasing the bone resorption.

Since osteoporosis disrupts bone quality, patients with osteoporosis are at increased risk of fractures. The BMD provides information on the likelihood of fracture risk in patients as lower is the BMD, higher is the risk of fracture and vice versa. Besides BMD, several factors identify the risk of fracture in an individual such as ageing, gender (post menopausal women), low body mass index, smoking, alcohol intake, parental history of hip fracture, previous fracture, steroid intake, rheumatoid arthritis and inflammatory bowel diseases.The risk of osteoporosis in general population is being assessed by fracture risk assessment tool (FRAX) provided by WHO [12].

Since osteoporosis is commonly seen in postmenopausal women or men above 50 years of age, this population group also has a high incidence of early CKD. Where as patients with late CKD have renal osteodystrophy, which is,characterized by abnormal bone quality with normal or high bone mineral content. Hence osteoporosis in CKD is most appropriate only for early CKD. Where as in CKD 4-5 or 5D stages (late CKD), low BMD should be designated as having 'CKD with low BMD.' The prevalence of osteoporosis is high in early CKD where as in late CKD it coexists with renal osteodystrophy.

1.3.2. CKD–MBD

KDIGO introduced a clear defined terminology for renal osteodystrophy in CKD patients, which is based on diagnostic tools [1].The wide spectrum of bone metabolic disorders, which, encompasses renal osteodystrophy is now defined as CKD associated mineral and bone disorder or CKD-MBD. This includes:

- Disruption in mineral homeostasis such as calcium, phosphorous
- Hormonal disturbances involving PTH, vitamin D and FGF-23
- Bone metabolic disorders characterized by high or low bone turnover affecting bone quality and strength
- Extra skeletal calcification (vascular or soft tissue) increasing the cardiovascular risk

Three types of bone metabolic disorders are seen in CKD-MBD as classified by bone histomorphometry:

- Osteitis fibrosa (OF): characterized by increased bone turnover and bone resorption due to secondary hyperparathyroidism
- Osteomalacia (OM): defective bone mineralization due to low vitamin D status
- Adynamic bone (ABD): reduced bone turnover characterized by reduced bone resorption and formation
- Mixed uremic osteodystrophy: characterized by mixed pattern of high and low bone turnover

CKD-MBD is usually seen inpatients with late CKD (stages 4-5/D). As CKD progresses to stage 3, mild secondary hyperparathyroidism results in high bone turnover where bone resorption exceeds bone formation. Further progress into stage 4 results in severe secondary hyperparathyroidism with markedly increased bone turnover manifesting as marrow fibrosis with increased osteoid production and abnormal mineralization. Further vitamin D deficiency due to reduced vitamin D production or resistance to its action in stage 4 leads to defective mineralization of bone or osteomalacia. Besides this, vitamin D deficiency also reduces the bone formation and increases the osteoclast production [13]. Approximately 60% of CKD-MBD present with normal or low bone turnover where as 40% present with high bone turnover.

Thus secondary hyperparathyroidism, which accompanies CKD, has a significant effect on the bone metabolism. Over the years, several approaches have been used to manage secondary hyperparathyroidism such as calcium salts to bind phosphate, vitamin D analogues to correct hypocalcaemia and vitamin D deficiency, parathyroidectomy in tertiary hyperparathyroidism to correct hypercalcaemia, calcimimetic drugs are used as an alternative to parathyroidectomy. All these therapies are given to reduce the effect of PTH on bone and therefore over-suppression of PTH over a prolonged time reduces the bone turnover and leads to adynamic bone disease (ABD) [14]. Studies have shown that 30% patients in CKD 4 and between 15 and 60% patients in CKD 5 or 5D has ABD [9]. ABD in CKD-MBD is characterized by subnormal osteoid tissue, mineralization, reduced osteoclast and osteoblast activity.Thus a large proportion of patients with CKD-MBD presents more frequently with ABD than OM or OF.

The prevalence of ABD has been increasing in CKD population. The exact mechanisms contributing to this type of bone disorders is largely unknown. Nevertheless, several factors are thought to be aggravating this type of low bone turnover renal osteodystrophy. Dialysis fluid containing aluminum is deposited in bone and can impair bone mineralization and reduce bone turnover. However aluminimum is no longer used in dialysis now. ABD is commonly seen in patients with diabetic nephropathy than in non-diabetics. Iron load is also thought to contribute to ABD. Patients with ABD are also susceptible to develop hypercalcaemia. Therisk of hypercalcaemia is exacerbated with administration of calcium carbonate in the CKD patients where it used as a phosphate binder. Patients with ABD have impaired ability to buffer calcium loads, a tendency to hypercalcaemia, as well as increased fracture rates and prevalence of extra-skeletal calcification.

1.3.3. Bone fragility fractures

Both osteoporosis and renal osteodystrophy in CKD-MBD can lead to increased bone fragility and fractures as both conditions are associated with low bone quality and poor bone microarchitecture. However both these diseases have different pathophysiological backgrounds. Bone fragility is due to varying combinations of low bone mineral content and abnormal bone quality. The fracture risk in CKD is magnified in elderly patients, women, diabetic, those using glucocorticoids, and in those with a longer exposure to dialysis. Patients in CKD are at higher risk of bone fragility fractures than those without CKD. FRAX (fracture risk assessment tool by WHO), which is used to estimate fracture risk in patients without CKD, is not applicable to patients with CKD as it will underestimate fracture risk.

The low impact fractures such as vertebral, non-vertebral and hip fractures are usually associated with osteoporosis as well as seen in CKD-MBD. The bone fragility fractures usually present with back pain leading to disability and death in these patients [15]. Hip fractures are common in CKD patients due to secondary hyperparathyroidism as PTH affects the cortical bone leading to high morbidity and mortality in these patients [16,17].

Patients with CKD-MBD have an increased risk of fracture compared with the general population, which can be due to osteomalacia, secondary hyperparathyroidism or adynamic bone.In CKD-MBD secondary hyperparathyroidism potentiates the risk of bone fractures by increasing the bone turnover as seen in OF and OM. ABD is presumed to increase the risk of bone fractures due to impair ability of bone to repair micro fractures due to low bone turnover.

2. Management of osteoporosis in CKD

Since CKD involves wide spectrum of bone metabolic disorders, the identification of osteoporosis from other bone metabolic disorders is essential particularly in late CKD stage.

2.1. Investigations

2.1.1. Bone Mineral density (BMD)

Patients in early CKD are diagnosed by bone mineral density measured by DEXA scan. BMD measurement is indicated in early CKD provided they do not have manifestations of CKD-MBD. Since CKD-MBD encompasses a wide spectrum of bone metabolic dystrophy, which varies from renal osteodystrophy to osteoporosis, BMD measurement by DEXA is unable to differentiate between the types of bone metabolic disorders. More importantly there is no evidence that BMD in CKD-MBD predict the fracture risk in this subpopulation unlike in patients with early CKD. The risk of fractures is high in CKD-MBD as compared to early CKD as both renal osteodystrophy and osteoporosis increases the risk of fractures.Thus, the routine use of BMD in patients with late CKDhas not been recommended. In patients with late CKD, the relationship between BMD and fractures is not as strong as that in the general population.

2.1.2. Biochemical markers

The biochemical markers are useful in assessing the bone metabolic status in CKD. These include:

- Hormones regulating the bone turnover
- Markers of bone collagen breakdown or formation
- Indicators of bone mineralization

The biochemical markers, help in differentiating the high bone turnover from low bone turnoverparticularly in CKD-MBD. Studies have shown that 40% CKD-MBD patients have high bone turnover compatible with OF and mixed bone disease where as 60% have low or normal bone turnover as seen in OM and AD.

Since these biochemical markers are non-specific they cannot help with the diagnosis of the type of bone metabolic disorder in CKD. They are helpful in monitoring the management of bone metabolic disorders in CKD patients.

- Hormones regulating the bone turnover

PTH regulates bone physiology. Serum PTH levels have been used as a surrogate indicator of bone turnover in the absence of bone biopsy.Raised PTH indicates vitamin D deficiency in early CKD where as late CKD it suggests high turnover bone metabolic disorders.PTH which is usually six times above the reference range, is associated with high bone turnover which can be seen in osteitis fibrosa cystica or osteomalacia but do not conclusively predict high turnover bone metabolic disease.The presence of low PTH (<15.9pmol/L or 150pg/ml) is consistent with low bone turnover osteodystrophy such as ABD. Thus raised PTH excludes the ABD in CKD-MBD.

- Biochemical markers of bone turnover

The markers of bone turnover help in the biochemical monitoring of bone metabolism. These markers include enzymes and proteins released during bone formation and degradation or resorption. The markers are not recommended for the diagnosis of osteoporosis. Nevertheless, they are useful in monitoring the treatment of osteoporosis in patients. The markers of bone turnover along with BMD are helpful in predicting the fracture risk in osteoporotic patients [18]. The markers are classified as formation markers, which are produced by osteoblasts or from pro collagen metabolism where as resorption markers are derived from degradation of osteoclasts or collagen tissue.

The markers of bone turnover includes:

a. Bone formation markers

  1. Bone Alkaline phosphatase (BALP)

  2. Type 1 N terminal procollagen peptide (P1NP)

  3. Type 1 C-terminal procollagen peptide (P1CP)

  4. Osteocalcin (OC)

b. Bone resorption markers

  1. C terminal telopeptide (CTX)

  2. N terminal telopeptide (NTX)

  3. Pyridinolines (PYR)

  4. Deoxypyridinolines (DPYR)

  5. Tartrate resistant acid phosphatase (TRACP)

Role of bone turnover markers in early CKD

In patients with early CKD, markers of bone turnover predict the status of bone metabolism.The biochemical status of bone turnover is monitored by release of proteins and enzymes during bone formation and degradation products during bone resoprtion. The bone turnover markers are associated with bone loss and this is more significant with bone resorption than formation markers [19]. Large observational studies have shown that bone turnover markers predict the fracture risk in osteoporotic patients and this is independent of BMD [20]. This relationship is again stronger for bone resorption than formation markers [21,22].

The bone turnover markers are not recommended for the diagnosis of osteoporosis as they have low specificity but high sensitivity in predicting the bone remodeling status. The bone turnover markers are recommended for the monitoring of therapy as they predict the response to treatment as early as 3-6months of starting therapy. Therefore bone turnover markers predict the changes in bone remodeling status much earlier than BMD. IOF (International Osteoporosis Foundation) and IFCC (International Federation of clinical chemistry) has produced the recommendation for using bone turnover markers in fracture risk prediction and monitoring of osteoporosis.

Among markers of bone resorption, CTX in blood is commonly used for predicting the bone resorption status where as serum P1NP is used commonly as marker of bone formation. Urinary markers such as PYR, DPYR are not used routinely due to problems associated with urine collection and is influenced by creatinine excretion.

In early CKD raised bone turnover markers suggest the presence of bone metabolic disorders such as osteoporosis, pagets, osteomalacia, recent fracture or bone metastasis. Besides this rise in bone resorption markers in osteoporoticpatients suggests:

- Risk of fractures
- Other bone metabolic diseases such as malignancy
- To initiate the treatment where BMD and clinical risk factors are not sufficient to make treatment decision

Osteoporotic patients on anti-resorptive therapy need repeat BMD every 2-3 years to assess the response to treatment. However, bone markers have the ability to assess the short-term response to anti-resorptive treatment every 6 monthly. Hence bone markers have a great value in monitoring ant-resorptive therapy in osteoporotic patients.

Among the markers of bone turnover, serum CTX or P1NP are preferred in monitoring the anti-resorptive treatment in osteoporotic patients with early CKD. The patients starting on anti-resorptive should have baseline serum CTX, treatment is monitored by evaluating the change in CTX at 6 month and reduction of >30% from baseline suggest efficacy and compliance to therapy [23].

Role of bone turnover markers in late CKD

Serum markers of bone remodeling can be useful to evaluate renal osteodystrophy in CKD-MBD.Most bone makers have renal metabolism and/or excretion and accumulate in renal failure.CTX, NTX, PYR and DPYR are influenced by renal function and its concentration in blood increases with deterioration in renal excretion. Among bone markers BALP, P1NP, P1CP and TRACP do not undergo renal metabolism or excretion and hence not influenced by renal functions.

The biochemical markers such as PTH and BALPare recommended for assessing the bone turnover in CKD-MBD. Further KDIGO does not suggest the use of markers of collagen degradation such as CTX/NTX or PYR/DPYR in late CKD. BALP is preferred over cross linked telopeptides (CTX/NTX) as it is not excreted or metabolized by kidney, assess the rate of bone formation and increased levels exclude the ABD [24]. Nevertheless, BALP is a non-specific marker of high bone turnover as raised BALP reflects bone metabolic disorders such as vitamin D deficiency, secondary hyperparathyroidism and recent fracture. BALP has emerged as one of the most sensitive marker of bone turnover and correlates with bone histomorphometry and BMD. Studies have shown that BALP is a useful bone marker in the diagnosis of ABD and low BALP has a high sensitivity and specificity in excluding ABD as compared to PTH [25]. Similarly raised PTH also reflects the high bone turnover, which predicts OF, OM and excludes ABD. BALP is a better predictor of bone turnover than PTH. Hence normal bone ALP with normal or elevated PTH excludes high bone turnover in CKD-MBD. Studies have shown that BALP ≥20U/L alone or with PTH ≥21pmol/L has the highest sensitivity, specificity, positive and negative predictive value for the diagnosis of high bone turnover and excludes patients with normal or low bone turnover [26].

There is minimal data on the bone turnover markers in predicting fracture risk in CKD-MBD patients. Several studies have shown that PTH and BALP are better markers of bone turnover in CKD-MBD patients [25,27].

Based on evidence available, raised BALP with or without raised PTH excludes ABD in CKD-MBD patients. This has been further endorsed by KDIGO, which recommends the use of BALP and PTH in assessing the bone status in CKD-MBD patients [28].

Recommendations:

i. Markers of bone turnover are non-specific markers of bone metabolism and therefore not to be used for the diagnosis of bone metabolic disorders in CKD.

ii. Markers of bone turnover are used in monitoring the efficacy of therapy in CKD.

iii. Serum CTX or P1NP are preferred makers for monitoring the therapy in osteoporotic patients in early CKD.

iv. Since BALP is not excreted by kidney, it is a useful marker of bone turnover in CKD-MBD

v. Low BALP indicates low bone turnover and ABD

vi. BALP above the reference range excludes ABD

vii. Besides BALP, TRACP is also not excreted by kidney and is a marker of increase bone resorption.

viii. PINP which is a marker of bone formation and not affected by reduced e GFR has not been investigated in CKD-MBD

ix. Bone resorption markers such as CTX are affected by reduced e GFR and thus not useful in evaluating the bone turnover status in CKD-MBD

x. BALP and PTH together increases the predictive value of identifying ABD in CKD-MBD

xi. Serum measurements of PTH and BALP are related to clinical outcomes, including relative risk of mortality. They also correlate with some of the bone histomorphometric measurements.

xii. The biochemical markers of bone turnover are non-invasive and convenient to measure unlike bone biopsy and can be used to assess the bone status in CKD-MBD

- Indicators of bone mineralization

The measurement of serum calcium, phosphorous and 25 (OH) vitamin D predict the status of bone mineralization in patients with CKD.

Serum calcium and phosphorous

The serum calcium is a poor predictor of total body calcium status as only 1% of calcium is extracellular and rest is in bone. The serum corrected calcium (after correcting serum calcium with albumin) is measured to assess the calcium status in clinical practice. Inorganic phosphorous plays a role in skeletal development. Serum phosphorous measures the inorganic phosphorous in blood. Both calcium and phosphorous are bound to hydroxyapatite crystals in bone, which helps with bone mineralization. Low serum calcium and phosphorous suggests vitamin D deficiency or secondary hyperparathyroidism. On the contrary, raised serum calcium or phosphorous in CKD patients suggest vitamin D over-replacement. The raised calcium and phosphorous in blood increases the risk of extra-skeletal calcification which further potentiates the cardiovascular risk in these patients. Thus monitoring of serum calcium and phosphorous is recommended in CKD patients particular in CKD-MBD patients.

Serum 25 (OH)vitamin D

Vitamin D deficiency is common in CKD patients due to impaired synthesis of active 1,25 (OH)D [29]. Low 25 (OH) vitamin D levels are seen in approximately 80% of patients with late CKD [26]. Studies have shown that 25 (OH) D has significant positive effect on PTH and BMD [30] as vitamin D deficiency aggravates the risk of secondary hyperparathyroidism, which further increases the bone resorption and bone metabolic disorders. Thus correction of vitamin D status has been recommended which will improve the bone mineralization.The serum 25 (OH) D above 75nmmol/L levels is recommended in CKD patients that will reduce the risk of secondary hyperparathyroidism and improve bone mineralization.

Recommendations:

- 25 (OH)D to be measured in patients with CKD to assess the bone mineral status
- 25 (OH)D should be above 75nmol/L in CKD patients
- Serum corrected calcium and phosphorous should be within the reference range

2.1.3. Bone biopsy

CKD–MBD can lead to an abnormal bone quality even in the setting of a normal or high bone-mineral content. Bone biopsy provides measurements of bone turnover, mineralization, and volume. These help to assess bone quality and the underlying bone physiology. Bone biopsy is a gold standard test for diagnosing the bone metabolic disorders in CKD-MBD. Nevertheless, it cannot be used in routine practice as it is a invasive procedure, painful to patient and can be carried out by an expert.Bone histomorphometery is studied by taking a biopsy from iliac crest of the bone. Since it is invasive procedure it cannot be carried routinely.

Recommendations:

- Bone biopsy is considered as the gold standard test for the diagnosis and classification of CKD-MBD.
- Not available routinely as it needs to be carried by a trained doctor.
- Bone biopsy is helpful if there is a history of unexplained bone pain or fracture in CKD-MBD patients to identify the type of bone metabolic disorder.

2.2. Treatment of bone metabolic disorders in CKD

Osteoporosis is a predominant bone metabolic disorder in early CKD where as its prevalence reduces in late CKD.

An osteoporotic patient in early CKD benefit with anti-resorptive treatment as it increases BMD and reduces fracture risk. Since CKD-MBD has wide spectrum of bone metabolic disorders, bisphosphonates may not be beneficial as seen in early CKD.The presence of ABD is a contraindication to bisphosphonates. In addition there is limited evidence regarding efficacy of treatments in reducing fracture risk in those patients with late CKD who have low BMD and biochemical abnormalities of CKD–MBD.

There are two types of therapies for treating osteoporosis in CKD: anti-resorptive which inhibits the osteoclastic induced bone resorption and anabolic therapy, which stimulates the osteoblastic induced bone formation.

Anti-resorptive is a first line therapy in the treatment of osteoporosis in postmenopausal women in whom it increases BMD both at cortical and trabecular site and reduces the fracture risk at vertebral, non-vertebral and hip.

Bisphosphonates (BP)

BP is the synthetic analogue of inorganic pyrophosphate, which inhibit the osteoclastic induced bone resorption and causes apoptosis of osteoclast. Thus BP reduces the bone turnover in osteoporosis. Alendronic acid is the commonly used BP and is recommended as first line therapy [31] for treating osteoporosis in post-menopausal women with osteoporosis. It has been shown to increase BMD and reduces the vertebral, non-vertebral and hip fractures.In early CKD patients with osteoporosis, BP is recommended as first line therapy. Recently continued use of BP in osteoporotic patients has been discouraged due to adverse affects associated with its long-term use. The risk of osteonecrosis of jaw and atypical fracture have been shown to be associated with prolonged use of BP. Hence it has been recommended to administer BP for 5 years in osteoporotic patients [32].

FDA and MHRA do not recommend the use of BP in patients with e GFR <30ml/min. Since BP have renal excretion, it may affect kidney function. Moreover, low BMD in CKD-MBD can be either due to renal osteodystrophy or osteoporosis, and therefore suggesting a cautious use of BP in this subpopulation of CKD.

Adminstration of BP in CKD-MBD patients with low bone turnover can have adverse consequences in the form of over-suppression leading to ABD. This will further increase the risk of fractures and extra-skeletal calcification increasing the morbidity in this group of patient.

2.2.1. Nephrotoxic effect of BP

There is a concern regarding nephrotoxic effect of BP. There is substantial evidence, which state that BP increases serum creatinine and this has been seen in cancer patients receiving intravenous bisphosphonate therapy.

BP administered intravenously does have nephrotoxic effect and intravenous zolendronic acid increases serum creatinine levels.Ibandronic acid may be less problematic in this respect. Approximately 50% of oral bisphosphonate is renally eliminated and the pharmacokinetics in renal impairment has not been fully elucidated.

Despite several reports, nephrotoxicity is uncommon and rarely of clinical significance when lower (osteoporotic range) doses of BP are used. Renal toxicity with BP appears to be associated with both dose and infusion time. Some experts recommend lower dose of BP to prevent nephrotoxicity. However there is lack of evidence related to effect of BP on fracture risk and BMD in CKD-MBD. Very few studies have assessed the effect of BP on renal function and have shown no difference in serum creatinine in patients administered BP over a period of three years in CKD 2-4 [33].Nevertheless, manufacturers do not recommend administration of BP in patients with e GFR less than 35ml/min in view of safety issues.

2.2.2. Effect of BP on bone turnover in CKD

The second area of concern relates to the skeleton itself. BP binds to hydroxyapatite and powerfully impairs resorptive activity, and thus reducing bone turnover rate. Since there are very few clinical trials involving small which have assessed the effect of BP on fracture risk in CKD-MBD, there is no clear evidence regarding its efficacy in this group of CKD. Therefore it is reasonable to administer BP only in those patients who have high bone turnover in CKD-MBD. However, BP need to be given cautiously in this group as they can reduce serum calcium levels by inhibiting bone resorption, thereby leading to secondary hyperparathyroidism which can be detrimental to bone. Additionally BP has a long retention time in bone, which can further induce parathyroid hyperplasia and can lead to adynamic bone. The incidence of ABD has increased in CKD patients particularly those on dialysis and BP administration can have deleterious effect. The risk of extra-skeletal calcification is high in ABD as it is associated with impaired ability of bone to buffer calcium. Moreover there is a increased risk of fracture in ABD which gets further aggravated by BP impairing the bone strength and quality.

Therefore patients with reduced bone turnover in CKD-MBD may benefit with anabolic therapy which will increase the bone formation. This will be a more logical approach in managing the bone metabolic disorder in CKD-MBD.

Hence the theoretical hypothesis does not favour the administration of BP in low bone turnover CKD-MBD.This implies that ideally bone biopsy should be performed before administration of BP in late CKD patients. However similar benefit might be obtained more simply by using indirect measures of biochemical markers of bone turnover such as BALP and PTH.

2.2.3. Extra-skeletal calcification

Vascular calcifications are a serious problem in patients with CKD-MBD. There has been suggestion that BP by reducing the bone turnover in CKD-MBD can exacerbate the risk of vascular calcification. The interaction between BP and vascular calcification is complexwhich is related to low bone turnover effect of BP. Several studies have shown that low bone turnover is unable to buffer calcium and phosphate load increasing the risk of vascular calcification [34]

2.2.4. Effect of BP on fracture risk

The patients with early CKD with no biochemical abnormalities will benefit from BP as shown in general population in terms of fracture prevention and risk [35,36].

The decision regarding BP use is more difficult in late CKD who present with bone mineral disorder and have been having fractures. Studies so far carried in late CKD are confined to stage 4, are post hoc analysis and have small sample size and thus difficult to interpret their results with regards to fracture risk in this sub-population [37].There are no published data for the safety and efficacy of BP in patients with CKD 5/5D.

Recommendations

- BP is recommended for the treatment of osteoporosis in early CKD
- BP use in late CKD can be detrimental than beneficial due to concerns, around its appropriateness and safety
- There is no reliable evidence regarding the efficacy of BP in late CKD
- Since BP have longer bone retention, it may exacerbate the risk of vascular calcification and atypical fractures in late CKD patients

Role of Denosumab (DN)

Denosumab, a receptor activator of nuclear factor kappa-B ligand (RANKL) inhibitor, is not cleared by the kidney and may be safe in patients with CKD. DN inhibits the bone resorption by reducing the production of osteoclasts, thereby increasing the BMD at both lumbar and hip and reducing the vertebral and hip fractures [38].

DN unlike BP is not metabolized or excreted by the kidney and does not affect kidney function [39].DN is recommended by FDA in patients with low eGFR. Since DN is metabolized by reticuloendothelial cells, it has a shorter duration of action lasting 3-6months and therefore shorter retention time in bone. Efficacy and safety of DN in reducing fracture risk has been demonstrated in post hoc studies in CKD stage 4 [40].Besides this it has a shorter retention time in bone [41]. Study by Jamal et al showed that DN significantly increased BMD and reduced fracture risk in postmenopausal women with CKD 1-4 [40].

Nonetheless, severe hypocalcaemia has been reported post DN in patients with late CKD or on dialysis [42]. It has been suggested that post DN therapy in CKD-MBD simulates the hungry bone syndrome. CKD-MBD is characterized by secondary hyperparathyroidism resulting in increased bone resorption. By giving DN in such patients there is inhibition of bone resorption, which promotes the bone uptake of calcium thereby causing severe hypocalcaemia. Thus patients with severe hyperparathyroidism with concomitant vitamin D deficiency are at potential risk of severe hypocalcaemia following DN [42].Recent MHRAalert Oct 2012, has reported the risk of hypocalcaemia in patients with e GFR<30ml/min.Therefore MHRA recommends the supplementation of calcium and vitamin D in such patients to avoid hypocalcaemia.

DN is considered to be safe in late CKD as it does not affect renal functions and has shorter bone retention time. There is no evidence that DN over suppresses the bone turnover and potentiates the risk of ABD in late CKD. However, it has been suggested to carry out bone biopsy before administration of DN in CKD 5/5D.

Recommendation

- DN is recommended for the management of osteoporosis in early CKD
- DN is safe to administer in late CKD as it neither affects kidney function nor metabolized by kidney
- It has a shorter duration of action and has shorter retention time in bone, therefore its affect on bone turnover will reverse after an interval of 6 months
- Post hoc studies have shown that it increases BMD and reduces the fracture risk in CKD 4, nevertheless there is no evidence regarding its efficacy on bone in CKD 5/5D

Strontium Ranelate in CKD

The mode of action of SR is thought to be dual with both anti-resorptive and mild anabolic. It is approved for the treatment of postmenopausal osteoporosis as it reduces the risk of vertebral and hip fractures. Nevertheless, it is not recommended for the treatment of osteoporosis in patients with late CKD. Its use in early CKD for the management of osteoporosis is contraindicated in patients with cardiovascular diseases, uncontrolled hypertension and deep venous thrombosis.

Raloxifene

Raloxifene is a selective estrogen receptor modulator and is approved for the management of osteoporosis in postmenopausal women. It reduces the risk of vertebral fractures but has not been shown to reduce the hip fractures. Its use is contraindicated in patients with late CKD.

Teriparatide

Teriparatide is a human recombinant hormone that contains amino acid residues 1-34 of the 84 amino acid sequence of human PTH. It is an anabolic agent that has been shown to improve the spine and hip BMD and reduces the vertebral and non-vertebral fracture [43]. It is approved for the treatment of postmenopausal osteoporosis in women and in men. It has been recommended to treat patients with severe osteoporosis with teriparatide who have been having recurrent fractures in spite of being on anti-resorptive treatment.

The safety and efficacy of teriparatide have been demonstrated in patients with early CKD (eGFR >30 mL/min), but there are no data on the use of this agent in patients with eGFR <30 mL/min. Teriparatide is contraindicated in patients with early CKD who have hypercalcaemia, elevated PTH, bone metabolic disorders other than osteoporosis and malignancy.

Calcium and vitamin D

In CKD patients with osteoporosis, calcium and vitamin D supplementation is recommended at the same dose as it is used for individuals with postmenopausal osteoporosis. Optimal calcium intake of 1200mg daily and optimal 25 (OH) D levels ≥75nmol/L are suggested by various guidelines. Vitamin D supplementation in the form of cholecalciferol or vitamin D analogues is approved for the treatment of postmenopausal osteoporosis. It has been shown to reduce the risk of vertebral fractures in postmenopausal women with osteoporosis.

2.2.5. Recommendations on the treatment of osteoporosis in CKD

- BP is the first line of osteoporosis treatmentin early CKD whereas it is not recommended for the treatment of low BMD in late CKD
- DN is safe to administer in late CKD
- DN should be given cautiously in late CKD as there is risk of hypocalcaemia and adynamic bone with its administration
- Adequate intake of calcium and vitamin D is important in patients with late CKD before DN therapy
- Before administration of DN, serum calcium should be within the reference range and 25 (OH) D levels should be ≥75nmol/L in late CKD

3. Critical appraisal of evidence

3.1. Kidney Disease – Improving Global Outcomes (KDIGO) published the recommendations for the management of osteoporosis and CKD-MBD in CKD patients

KDIGO Clinical Practice Guidelines for the diagnosis, evaluation, prevention and treatment of Chronic Kidney Disease – Mineral and Bone Disorder (CKD-MBD) (Kidney Int. 2009; vol 76 suppl 113, s1-132]

Following are the recommendations made by KDIGO 2009 guideline in managing CKD-MBD

- The bone biopsy and histological/histomorphometric diagnosis is helpful in classification of CKD-MBD
- It is reasonable to perform a bone biopsy in various settings including: unexplained fractures, persistent bone pain, unexplained hypercalcaemia, unexplained hypophospha-

temia, possible aluminum toxicity, and prior to anti-resorptive therapy in patients with osteoporosis

- BMD does not predict fracture in CKD-MBDand should not be used routinely
- Serum 25 (OH) D should be measured routinelyand corrected
- Monitor serum levels of calcium, phosphorus, PTH, and alkaline phosphatase activity
- Measurements of serum PTH or BALP can be used to evaluate bone disease because markedly high or low values predict underlying bone turnover
- Routine measurement of bone-derived turnover markers of collagen synthesis such as P1CP/P1NP and breakdown such as CTX, NTX, PDY, DPYD is not recommended
- Patients with levels of intact PTH above the upper normal limit of the assay need to be evaluated for hyperphosphatemia, hypocalcaemia, and vitamin D deficiency
- It is reasonable to correct these abnormalities with any or all of the following: reducing dietary phosphate intake and administering phosphate binders, calcium supplements, vitamin D supplements and calcimimetics
- In patients with persistently high serum PTH, treatment with calcitriol or vitamin D analogs is suggested
- In patients with CKD stage 5D, maintaining PTH levels in the range of approximately two to nine times the upper normal limit for the assay

3.2. Suggested protocol for management of osteoporosis in CKD

CKD 1-3 (early CKD)

- DEXA: T scores suggest osteoporosis
- Treat as postmenopausal osteoporosis

CKD 4-5 /dialysis (e GFR ≤30 or late CKD)

- DEXA not helpful in predicting osteoporosis and does not predict fracture risk
- Bone fragility fracture can be due to renal osteodystrophy/ osteoporosis
- Biochemical markers: BALP and PTH may be used to assess the bone turnover

Increased bone turnover

Raised BALP and PTH

- Exclude other causes of raised bone markers before treating high bone turnover:
  - Vitamin D deficiency
  - Hypocalcaemia
  - Hyperphosphatemia

http://dx.doi.org/10.5772/59607

If any of THE above present than correct and recheck BALP and PTH

- If vitamin D sufficiency (≥75nmol/L) WITH serum adjusted calcium and serum phosphate levels within the reference range
  - Administer Denosumab 60mg subcutaneous
  - Monitor BALP after therapy every 6 months
  - Administer further Denosumab only if there is a rise in BALP

Reduced bone turnover

Normal BALP and normal PTH/mildly elevated PTH

- No treatment with anti-resorptive therapy

4. Summary

Osteoporosis in early CKD is treated similar to general population. In late CKD or CKD-MBD, it is difficult to identify the type of bone metabolic disorder. Moreover, treatment of bone metabolic disorders is complicated by mineral and hormonal disturbances seen in late CKD. Also, there is a high prevalence of ABD in CKD-MBD and administration of anti-resorptive potentiates the risk of ABD or vascular calcification. Hence judicious use of anti-resorptive therapy is required in late CKD.

Following protocol can be followed for the management of Osteoporosis in late CKD or CKD-MBD:

- There are no published data on the safety and efficacy of any approved agent for osteoporosis among men and women with eGFR <30 or in late CKD
- In clinical practice, at the current time and with current limited knowledge, treatment of osteoporosis in stage 4-5/D CKD or late CKD is opinion based
- A reasonable clinical approach would be to consider therapy only in those with bone fragility fractures
- After exclusion of ABD (low bone turnover) and osteomalacia (vitamin D deficiency); high bone turnover should be considered for treatment with anti-resorptive therapy
- Osteoporosis in CKD-MBD is a diagnosis of exclusion
- Correct the biochemical abnormalities associated with CKD-MBD i.e. calcium and phosphate within the reference range; optimal vitamin D levels (≥75nmol/L)
- Increased bone turnover is indicated by: raised BALP after correction of calcium, phosphate and vitamin D levels (as mentioned above)
- Avoid DEXA: poor association of BMD with fracture risk

- Low BMD is not an indicator of treatment with anti-resorptive therapy
- Denosumab is the preferred treatment and should be administered after correcting calcium and vitamin D status
- Avoid Denosumab in severe hyperparathyroidism (>30pmol/L) as there is a risk of hypocalcaemia
- Post Denosumab therapy: check BALP every 6 monthly to assess the response to treatment
- Administer Denosumab only if there is rise in BALP

Author details

Vinita Mishra*

Address all correspondence to: vinita.mishra@rlbuht.nhs.uk

Clinical Biochemistry and Metabolic Medicine, Royal Liverpool and Broadgreen University, Hospital NHS Trust, Liverpool, UK

The aim of this article will be to critically analyse the evidence available with regards to management of osteoporosis in chronic kidney diseases (CKD)

References

[1] National Kidney Foundation. K/DOQI clinical practice guidelines for chronic kidney disease: Evaluation, classification, and stratification. *Am J Kidney Dis.* 2002;39 (2 suppl 1):S1-S266.

[2] KDIGO 2012 Clinical Practice Guideline for
the Evaluation and Management of Chronic Kidney Disease. *Kidney Int.* 2013;3 (suppl):1–150.

[3] Levin A, Bakris GL, Molitch M, et al. Prevalence of abnormal serum vitamin D, PTH, calcium, and phosphorus in patients with chronic kidney disease: results of the study to evaluate early kidney disease. *Kidney Int.* 2007;71:31–38.

[4] Jüppner H, Wolf M, Salusky IB. FGF-23: more than a regulator of renal phosphate handling? *J Bone Miner Res.* 2010;25:2091–2097.

[5] Fukumoto S, Yamashita T. FGF23 is a hormone-regulating phosphate metabolism – unique biological characteristics of
FGF23. *Bone.* 2007;40:1190–1195.

[6] Kazama JJ, Sato F, Omori K, Hama H, Yamamoto S, Maruyama H, Narita I, Gejyo F, Yamashita T, Fukumoto S, Fuka- gawa M: Pretreatment serum FGF-23 levels predict the effi- cacy of calcitriol therapy in dialysis patients. *Kidney Int* 2005; 67: 1120–1125.

[7] Slatopolsky E, Finch J, Denda M, et al. Phosphorus restriction prevents parathyroid gland growth. High phosphorus directly stimulates PTH secretion in vitro. *J ClinInvest.* 1996;97:2534–2540.

[8] Martin KJ, Gonzalez EA, Slatopolsky E: The parathyroids in renal disease: Pathophysiology. In: *The Parathyroids: Basic Clinical Concepts,* 2nd edition, San Diego, Academic Press Inc., 2001, pp 625– 634.

[9] Malluche HH, Mawad HW, Monier-Faugere MC. Renal osteodystrophy in the first decade of the new millennium: analysis of 630 bone biopsies in black and white patients. *J Bone Miner Res.* 2011; 26:1368–1376.

[10] Jan de Beur SM. Tumor-induced osteomalacia. *JAMA.* 2005; 294:1260–1267.

[11] Office of the Surgeon General (US). *Bone Health and Osteoporosis: A Report of the Surgeon General.* Rockville (MD): Office of the Surgeon General (US); 2004.

[12] Kanis JA on behalf of the World Health Organization Scientific Group. *Assessment of osteoporosis at the primary health care level.* Technical Report. World Health Organization Collaborating Center for Metabolic Bone Diseases. University of Sheffield, UK; 2007.

[13] Baldock PA, Thomas GP, Hodge JM, et al. Vitamin D action and regulation of bone remodeling: suppression of osteoclastogenesis by the mature osteoblast. *J Bone Miner Res.* 2006;21:1618–1626.

[14] Haris A, Sherrard DJ, Hercz G. Reversal of adynamic bone disease by lowering of dialysate calcium. *Kidney Int.*
2006;70:931–937.

[15] Lewiecki EM, Laster AJ. Clinical review: Clinical applications of vertebral fracture assessment by dual-energy x- ray absorptiometry. *J Clin Endo Metab.* 2006;91 (11): 4215-4222.

[16] Jamal SA, Hayden JA, Beyene J. Low bone mineral density and fractures in long-term hemodialysis patients: a meta- analysis. *Am J Kidney Dis.* 2007;49:674–681.

[17] Leinau L, Perazella MA. Hip fractures in end-stage renal disease patients: incidence, risk factors, and prevention. *Semin Dial.* 2006;19:75–79.

[18] Brown JP, Albert C, Nassar BA, Adachi JD, Cole D, Davison KS, et al. Bone turnover-markers in the management of postmenopausal osteoporosis. *Clin Biochem.* Aprl 2009;42 (10-11):929-42.

[19] Rosen CJ, Chesnut CH III and Mallinak NJ. The pre- dictive value of biochemical markers of bone turnover for bone mineral density in early postmenopausal women

treated with hormone replacement or calcium supplementation. J Clin Endocrinol Metab 1997; 82: 1904–1910

[20] Meier C, Nguyen TV, Center JR, et al. Bone resorption and osteoporotic fractures in elderly men: the Dubbo osteoporosis epidemiology study. J Bone Miner Res 2005; 20: 579–587

[21] Garnero P, Cloos P, Sornay-Rendu E, et al. Type I collagen racemization and isomerization and the risk of frac- ture in postmenopausal women: the OFELY prospective study. J Bone Miner Res 2002; 17: 826–833.

[22] Garnero P, Sornay-Rendu E, Claustrat B, et al. Biochemical markers of bone turnover, endogenous hor- mones and the risk of fractures in postmenopausal women: the OFELY study. J Bone Miner Res 2000; 15: 1526–1536

[23] Eastell R, Bauman M, Hoyle NR, Wieczorek L, eds. *Bone Markers: Biochemical and Clinical Perspectives.* London: Martin Dunitz Ltd; 2001.

[24] Brandenburg VM, Floege J. Adynamic bone disease – bone and beyond. *NDT Plus.* 2008;3:135–147.

[25] Couttenye M, P D'Haese P, VanHoof V, et al. Low serum levels of alkaline phosphatase of bone origin: a good marker of adynamic bone disease in haemodialysis patients. *Nephrol Dial Transpl.* 1996;11:1065–72.

[26] Barreto FC, Barreto DV, Moysés MA, et al. K/DOQI-recommended intact PTH levels do not prevent low-turnover bone
disease in hemodialysis patients. *Kidney Int.* 2008;73:771–777.

[27] Bervoets AR, Spasovski GB, Behets GJ, et al. Useful biochemical markers for diagnosing renal osteodystrophy in predialysis end- stage renal failure patients. *Am J Kidney Dis*. 2003;41 (5):997– 1007.

[28] Kidney Disease Improving Global Outcomes (KDIGO) CKD- MBD Work Group. KDIGO clinical practice guideline for the diagnosis, evaluation, prevention, and treatment of chronic kidney disease-mineral and bone disorder (CKD-MBD*). Kidney Int*. 2009;76 suppl 113:s1–130.

[29] González EA1, Sachdeva A, Oliver DA, Martin KJ.Vitamin D insufficiency and deficiency in chronic kidney disease. A single center observational study.*Am J Nephrol.* 2004 Sep-Oct;24 (5):503-10.

[30] Tomida K1, Hamano T, Mikami S, Fujii N, Okada N, Matsui I, Nagasawa Y, Moriyama T, Ito T, Imai E, Isaka Y, Rakugi H. Serum 25-hydroxyvitamin D as an independent determinant of 1-84 PTH and bone mineral density in non-diabetic predialysis CKD patients.*Bone* 2009 Apr;44 (4):678-83.

[31] Kanis JA, Adams J, Borgstrom F, Cooper C, Jönsson B Preedy D, Selby P, Compston J. The cost-effectiveness of alendronate in the management of osteoporosis. *Bone* 2008;42: 4-15.

[32] Black DM, Bauer DC, Schwartz AV et al. Continuing bisphosphonate treatment for osteoporosis – for whom and for how long? *New Engl J Med* 2012;366:2051-3.

[33] Miller PD, Roux C, Boonen S et al. *J Bone Miner Res* 2005; 20:2105–2115.

[34] Susan M. Ott. Bisphosphonate safety and efficacy in chronic kidney disease.*Kidney International* (2012) 82: 833-835.

[35] National Institute for Health and Clinical Excellence. Final appraisal determination. Alendronate, etidronate, risedronate, raloxifene, strontium ranelate and teriparatide for the secondary prevention of osteoporotic fragility fractures in postmenopausal women. London, *NICE*. June 2007.

[36] National Institute for Health and Clinical Excellence. Final appraisal determination. Alendronate, etidronate, risedronate, raloxifene, strontium ranelate and teriparatide for the secondary prevention of osteoporotic fragility fractures in postmenopausal women. London, *NICE*. June 2007.

[37] Jamal SA, Bauer DC, Ensrud KE, et al. Alendronate treatment in women with normal to severely impaired renal function: an anal- ysis of the fracture intervention trial. *J Bone Miner Res*. 2007;22 (4):503–8.

[38] Cummings SR, San Martin J, McClung MR, et al. Denosumab for prevention of fractures in postmenopausal women with osteoporosis. *N Engl J Med*. 2009;361:756–765.

[39] Boyle WJ, Simonet WS, Lacey DL. Osteoclast differentiation and activation. *Nature*. 2003;423:337–342.

[40] Jamal SA, Ljunggren O, Stehman-Breen C, et al. Effects of denosumab on fracture and bone mineral density by level of kidney function. *J Bone Miner Res*. 2011;26 (8): 1829–35.

[41] Delmas PD. Clinical potential of RANKL inhibition for the management of postmenopausal osteoporosis and other metabolic bone diseases. *J Clin Densitom*. 2008;11:325–338.

[42] Block GA, Bone HG, Fang L, Lee E, Padhi D. A singledose study of denosumab in patients with various degrees of renal impairment. *J Bone Miner Res*. 2012;27:1471–1479.

[43] Miller PD, Schwartz EN, Chen P, Misurski DA, Krege JH. Teriparatide in postmenopausal women with osteoporosis and mild or moderate renal impairment. Osteoporos Int. 2007;18:59–68.

Chapter 8

Hydrophilic Matrix Tablets Based on Carbopol for Improving the Oral Bioavailability of Sodium Alendronate — *In vitro* and *In vivo* Assessment

Lacramioara Ochiuz, Anca Giorgiana Grigoras and
Cristina Mihaela Ghiciuc

Additional information is available at the end of the chapter

http://dx.doi.org/10.5772/59510

1. Introduction

Sodium alendronate (hereinafter, AL-Na) is one of the most important drug substances of the bisphosphonate class administered orally for the treatment of all types of osteoporosis. Alendronate has a positive influence on all symptoms of osteoporosis by increasing bone mineral density and pacient mobility, reducing the risk of osteoporotic fractures in all vulnerabilities (vertebrae, hip, arm and femoral neck) and having an analgesic effect in bone pain. The anti-resorptive mechanism of action of AL-Na is complex and involves effects at both the molecular and the cellular level. Osteoclasts and their precursors are the target cells of AL-Na and, by internalization, they absorb the AL-Na molecule from the surface of bone. At the molecular level, AL-Na prevents the conversion of dimethyl-allyl pyrophosphate to geranyl - geranyl - pyrophosphate. Besides the biochemical effects described above, AL-Na also produces a number of effects at the cellular level, among which loss of brush border and fractures in the osteoclast cytoskeleton. All these actions of AL-Na ultimately lead to an increase in bone mineral density and to osteoclast-mediated inhibition of bone resorption. It is important to note that the anti-resorptive effect of AL-Na occurs the day after the first dose, the intensity of the therapeutical effect being directly dependent on the active substance dose administered [1, 2]. The results of the Fosamax Fracture Intervention Trial Long-term Extension (FLEX) showed that patients treated with AL-Na for 5 years presented an obvious increase in bone mineral density in the femoral neck, as well as in the lumbar spine. The results of this 10-year study showed a 17.7% decrease in the risk of vertebral fracture compared with placebo [3, 4]. Currently, AL-Na is used in daily (10 mg/tablet) or weekly (70 mg/tablet with or without

2 800 I.U. of vitamin D_3) conventional release tablets. Tablets with a higher concentration of vitamin D3 (70 mg AL-Na/5600 IU cholecalciferol/tablet) have also been introduced in therapy quite recently [5]. The exogenous intake of cholecalciferol contributes to the normalization of calcium homeostasis in the body and to the optimization of the anti-resorptive effect caused by AL-Na. Furthermore, it is known that a low level of vitamin D3 manifests in muscle weakness which can cause accidents with high risk of fracture [6].Once-weekly administered tablets (70 mg/tablet) have largely increased patient compliance with alendronate and led to a reduction in the incidence of gastrointestinal side effects. Pharmacokinetic studies have shown that oral doses of alendronate in the range 5-80 mg generate a bioavailability of 0.1-1%, with a fraction of 50% of the amount deposited in the bone. In addition, it was shown that oral administration of 10 mg alendronate daily and of 70 mg alendronate once-weekly generates the same level of increase in bone mineral density: 5-6% in the vertebrae and 3-9% in the femoral bone. Alendronate administered orally in the form of a solution (70 mg/vial) is intended for patients with deficiencies in swallowing. The latest alendronate formulation approved by Food and Drug Administration (FDA) and European Medicines Evaluation Agency (EMEA) is the association of 70 mg alendronate with 2800 I.U. vitamin D in immediate release tablets [7, 8]. According to FDA guidelines, there is no deadline or optimal duration for the treatment with AL-Na. The treatment with AL-Na is recommended for as long as necessary along with regular reassessment of patients (at intervals of no longer than five years) in order to determine bone mineral density and fracture risk [9].

However, low oral bioavailability (under 1%) is the most important disadvantage of AL-Na. It is caused by several factors such as: low permeability due to its negatively charged molecules (AL belongs to the 3rd class of biopharmaceutical classification system); short plasma half-time ($T_{½}$ = 0.5-2 h); its chelatation by Ca^{2+} ions resulting in non-absorbable complexes. Research in bisphosphonates in general aims *to increase the bioavailability of these substances, to decrease side effects, to increase adherence to treatment* especially for elderly patients. AL-Na has been in the attention of drug researchers and literature has presented a large number of studies on this topic. Investigations conducted in the formulation of alendronate sodium are directed to conventional pharmaceutical forms (solutions, emulsions, gels) as well as to modified-release forms (matrix tablets, microemulsions, micro– and nanoparticulate drug delivery systems) administered on various routes (Table 1).

In this study we have investigated the possibility of improving the oral bioavailability of AL-Na by including it in hydrophilic matrix tablets based on various sorts of Carbopol. The role of chitosan (CHT) and trimethyl chitosan (TMC) as AL-Na absorption enhancers was also researched.

Carbopol polymers form an important class of excipients used for the formulation and preparation of sustained release hydrophilic matrix tablets. Carbopols were synthesized and patented in 1957 [24]. Since then, a variety of therapeutic agents (such as the agents in the 3rd group of the biopharmaceutical system of drug classification: atenolol, verapamil, theophylline, metoprolol, ranitidine, etc.) have been formulated and prepared in different Carbopol-based formulations with controlled release [25-30].

Administration route	Pharmaceutical dosage form	References
Oral route	*Modified-release tablets:* 1. *HPMC-based matrix tablets* with different degrees of viscosity;	[10]
	2. *Gastro-resistant tablets* using various sorts of ethyl cellulose and acrylic derivatives as coating agents(Aquacoat ECD, Eudragit L30, Eudragit L-30-D55)	[11]
	Effervescent tablets	[12, 13]
	Solutions	[14]
	H/L Microemulsions with Captex 200 ® and lecithin as emulsifier	[15]
	Microparticulate therapeutic systems based on Eudragit S100/HPMC PLGA	[16-18]
Gingival-dental mucosa	*Carbopol-based gels*	[19]
Vaginal mucosa	*HPMC-based gels*	[20]
Nasal mucosa	*Microparticulate therapeutic systems based on* HPMC as unique excipient or associated with PVP	[21]
Transcutaneous	*Reservoir-type transdermal therapeutic systems* based on acrylic polymers in combination with various percutaneous absorption promoters: lauric acid, oleic acid, linoleic acid, myristic acid	[22]
	Gels prepared with different sorts of Duro-Tak® (acrylic acid copolymers) using propylene glycol and fatty acids as absorption promoters (lauric acid, oleic acid, linoleic acid and myristic) at various concentrations	[23]

Table 1. Examples of studies focused on increasing AL-Na bioavailability

From the chemical point of view, Carbopols are crosslinked polymers of acrylic acid (Figure 1), insoluble in water, characterized by a high degree of hydration.

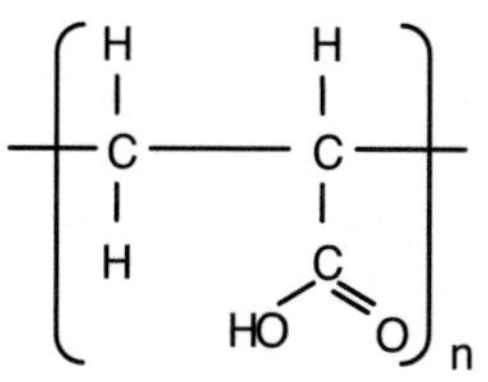

Figure 1. General chemical structure of Carbopol polymers

According to the literature, Carbopol polymers generally exhibit good compressibility characteristics, and this achieves compression at low pressures; are compatible with other matrix forming hydrophilic agents and many excipients; may help mask taste and have bioadhesive properties [31].

In the formulations studied, we used three Carbopol sorts with different crosslinking degrees: Carbopol 971 C (C 971), Carbopol 71 C (C 71) and Carbopol 974 C (C 974). These polymers are obtained by the crosslinking reaction of acrylic acid with allyl penta erythrol, followed by a polymerization reaction in ethyl acetate and neutralization with aqueous potassium hydroxide 1-3%. Although C 971 and C 974 are obtained by a similar technological process, the difference is that sort C 971 has a lower level of crosslinking agent compared to C 974. C 71 is the granular form of C 971 recommended to be used in direct compression [32-34]. Unlike the hydrophilic linear polymers soluble in polar solvents, whose absorption capacity is dependent on molecular weight, crosslinked Carbopol polymers are insoluble in water, since crosslinking degree is the determinant parameter of he matrix absorption capacity [35-37].

2. Investigations on the influence of carbopol sort on the release of alendronate sodium from modified release matrix tablets

Prior to this research, in our department of Pharmaceutical Technology we have also studied the influence of the concentration of Carbopol on the hydration and erosion characteristics of matrices in order to establish the optimal conditions for the development of these formulations [38-40]. Based on these results, in the present study we introduced 15% hydrophilic matrix forming polymer in the formulation. We used three sorts of Carbopol with different crosslinking degrees as matrix generating polymers: C 71 to C 971, polymers with a low of crosslinking degree, and C 974, a Carbopol with a high crosslinking degree. The research conducted has been focused on investigating the influence of the Carbopol sort on the release of alendronate from modified release matrix tablets.

2.1. Materials and methods

2.1.1. Materials

Alendronate sodium trihydrate (Apotex Pharmaceutics INC, USA), Carbopol 974 P NF, 971 P NF, 71 G NF (Noveon Inc.), Ludipress LCE (BASF), Aerosil 200 (Degussa), Magnesium stearate (Union Derlivan S.A. Spain).

2.1.2. Methods

2.1.2.1. Preparation of matrix tablets

Three formulations of alendronate sodium matrix tablets were prepared by the method of direct compression in the Korsh EK0 tablet machine (punch diameter of 9 mm, 8 to 10 kN compression force). As matrix forming polymer, formulations denoted F1, F2, F3 contain, as follows: 15% C 71 in F1, 15% C 971 in F2, and a mixture of 15:2% C 971:C974 – 15:2% in F3 (Table 2).

http://dx.doi.org/10.5772/59510

Ingredients (mg %)	Formulation		
	F1	F2	F3
C 71	15	–	–
C 971	–	15	15
C 974	–	–	2
AL-Na	13.05	13.05	13.05
Mg Stearate	0.5	0.5	0.8
Aerosil	–	0.5	1.5
Ludipress LCE	71.45	70.95	67.65

Table 2. Formulations of matrix tablets with AL modified release based on Carbopol

2.1.2.2. "In vitro" dissolution investigations

"In vitro" dissolution tests were carried out on a *SR 8 Plus Series* (AB & L Jasco) device, under the following experimental protocol: *dissolution medium*: pH 1.2 solution (0.1 N HCl) for the first 2 hours (a medium simulating gastric fluids) and solution pH 6.8 (phosphate buffer solution) for the next 10 hours (a medium simulating intestinal fluids); *Apparatus 2 (paddle)*; *bath temperature*: 37ºC±0.5 ºC; *rotation speed*: 50 rpm; sampling interval was set to every hour during the 12 hours of the test (at every collection, 7 ml of sample were replaced with the same volume of medium).

One sample from the aliquot was subjected to the derivation and dosage procedure described in the USP monography for the HPLC analysis of sodium alendronate. The quantitative determination equipment included the following modules: HPLC type HP 1090 series II provided with a diode array detector, UV-VIS spectrophotometer Agilent technologies 8453 and Zorbax C18 column. The mobile phase was a mixture of methanol, acetonitrile and water in the following proportions: 17.5:17.5:65. Mobile phase flow was set at 0.3 mL/min., the injection volume was 20μL and the detection was performed at 266 nm [41]. All the experiments were performed in triplicate.

Quantitative data were presented as mean ± standard deviation and statistical analysis was performed using a one-way analysis of variance (one-way ANOVA). A comparison between two means was made using Tukey's test, with statistical significance set at $p < 0.05$.

2.1.2.3. The analysis of the difference factor (f_1) and the similarity factor (f_2)

The two factors assessing the AL release profile in the investigated formulations were calculated according to the following equation:

$$f_1 = \left\{ \frac{\sum_{f-1}^{n} |R_t - T_t|}{\sum_{t-1}^{n} R_t} \right\} \times 100 \quad (1)$$

$$f_2 = 50\log_{10}\left\{\left[1+\frac{1}{n}\sum_{t-1}^{n}(R_t - T_t)2\right]^{-0.5}\times 100\right\} \tag{2}$$

where: n = the number of sampling time points, R_t = released AL percentage of the reference formula at time point t, T_t = released AL percentage of the test at time point t and $\log_{10}x$ represents the logarithm of x to the base 10 [42].

Difference factor f_1 is a measure for quantifying the differentiation degree of the release profile followed by a drug substance in the formulation. The value of this factor is in the interval 0 - 50. The analogy degree varies inversely with f_1 value. Thus, a value closer to 0 indicates a high similarity between two or more compared formulations. When the dissolution profile between the tested and the reference formula is identical, f_1 is 0 and increases with the dissimilarity between the formulas analyzed. In general, the values of the f_1 factor in the range 0-15 correspond to very small differences between the formulations tested, while values greater than 15 indicate major differences in the release profiles of the drug substances in the compared formulations.

Similarity factor f_2 is a parameter commonly used to compare the dissolution profiles of the solid oral pharmaceutical forms.

When two dissolution profiles of the drug substance are similar, f_2 is in the range of 50-100 [43, 44]. According to the FDA guidelines in force, the values of the f_2 similarity factor included between 50 and 100 show a high degree of similarity (≥ 90%) between the release profiles of the tested formulation against the reference formulation. Theoretically, values of the similarity factor f_2 smaller than 50 are accepted in the interpretation of the *in vitro* dissolution tests. Mention should be made that these values show a similarity <90% between the formulas analyzed.

Note that these two parameters are accepted and recommended by international quality guidelines for the comparative evaluation of the release profile of two or more formulations compared to a reference formulation, as can be seen in equations 1 and 2. While EMEA has not issued any regulations on the determination and analysis of difference factor f_1 and similarity factor f_2, FDA and USP regulate the applicability of these factors for the comparison of the release profile of two or more pharmaceutical formulations by the following clarifications: 1. release profiles between two or more formulas can be compared only when the dissolution test includes a minimum of 12 sampling points; 2 the conditions of the *in vitro* dissolution test should be identical for the reference formulation and for the tested formulations [45-47].

2.2. Results and discussions

Figure 2 presents the results obtained from the *in vitro* dissolution test for the studied formulations.

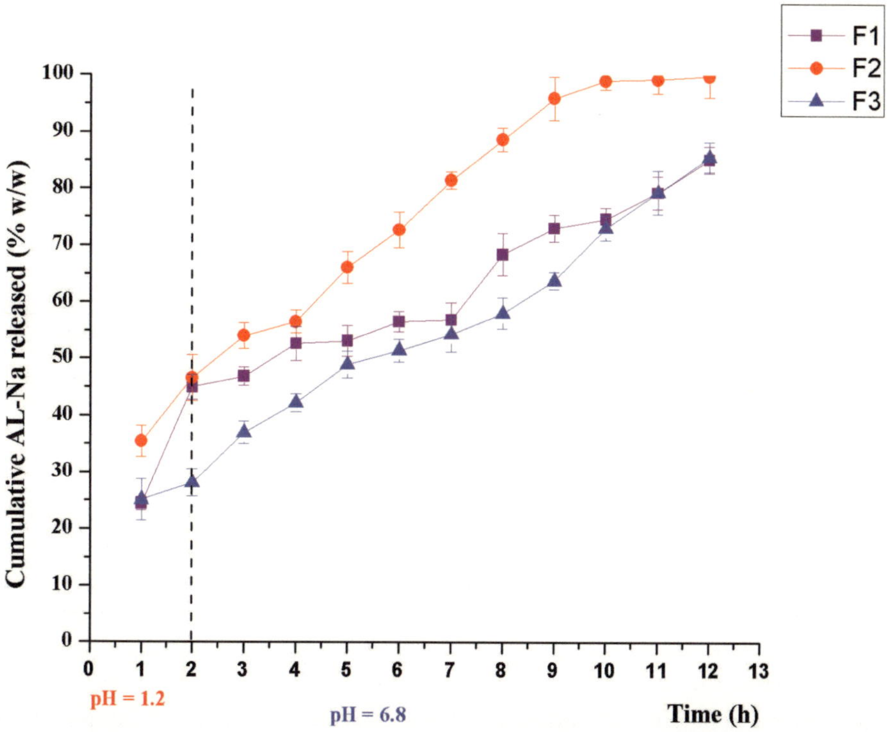

Figure 2. *In vitro* dissolution profile for AL in hydrophilic matrix tablets based on Carbopol

We can see from the results obtained that the dissolution profile of alendronate sodium in formulation F2 based on C 971 is superior to other formulations (99.7889% AL-Na released; t = 12 hours). In theory this result was not foreseeable because C 71 and C 971, the polymers in formulas F1 and F2, have the same degree of crosslinking, sort C71 actually having flow properties optimized by the granular particle form.

The influence of the crosslinking degree of the polymer in the formulation was also highlighted by the pH value of the dissolution medium. Thus, at acidic pH 1.2 simulating gastric fluids, C 71 and C 971, which are polymers with a low degree of crosslinking, showed a uniform hydration resulting in a uniform release of alendronate sodium in the matrix gel layers.

C 974, a polymer with a high degree of crosslinking, optimizes the retardation effect at gastric level through the closely crosslinked gel structure which acts as an element that reduces the diffusion of the drug substance in the hydrated matrix layers during the first hours of the test and accelerates this process after the total hydration of the matrix.

Finally, after performing the dissolution test within 12 hours, we found that the dissolution profile of alendronate sodium is identical in F1, the formula based on C 71, and in F3, the formula in which we associated C 974 as well (F1 = 85.1128% AL-Na released; F3 = 85.5984% AL-Na released), specifying that sort C 974 generates a slow dissolution profile within the first two hours of the test, at pH 1.2 (F1 = 44.9356% Na released; F2 = 46.5233% AL-Na released, F3 = 28.0566% AL-Na released, t = 2 hours).

The different behavior as regards the dissolution profile of alendronate sodium in modified release matrix tablets is also confirmed by the results obtained in the determination of f_1, the difference factor, and f_2, the similarity factor (Table 3).

Reference formula (R_t)	Test formula (T_t)	f_1	f_2
F1	F2	25.149	37.041
F1	F3	12.608	***50.940***
F2	F3	26.9546	34.1921

Table 3. Values of f_1 and f_2 factors obtained in the comparative analysis F1-F3

In the comparative analysis of the three formulations studied, the difference factor f_1 has values > 0. The similarity factor f_2, which is the most representative for the comparison of the dissolution profile of solid dosage forms also has values that indicate a different dissolution profile for the three formulations investigated (f_2 <50), with the exception of the comparison F1, reference, F3, test, when f_2 = 50, 940. We estimate that this value is determined by the evolution of the release pattern of AL-Na towards the end of the *in vitro* dissolution test, in 6.8 buffer system because there were no significant differences between the two formulas during the first two hours of the test, under conditions of simulated gastric fluid.

2.3. Conclusions

The results of the *in vitro* dissolution test reveal that every sort of Carbopol influences the release profile of alendronate sodium in matrix tablets with modified release. The crosslinking degree of Carbopol is the defining element of the release properties of hydrophilic matrix tablets. Sorts C 71 and C 971, with a low degree of crosslinking, hydrate much better at pH 1.2, a phenomenon which facilitates the dissolution of alendronate sodium, its diffusion through the gel layers of the matrix, and therefore, the release of a greater amount of drug substance compared to formula F3, in which we associated C 974, a high crosslinking polymer, which causes a slowing of the hydration process. The influence of the crosslinking degree of Carbopol also manifests at pH 6.8; F2, the formula based on C 971, generated a release profile of AL-Na superior to formula F3, in which we associated C 974 and C 971, and to formula F1 based on C 71, respectively.

The different dissolution profile of alendronate sodium in modified release matrix tablets based on Carbopol is further confirmed by the values of the two control parameters f_1 and f_2. The similarity factor f_2 is set to 50.940, little over 50, the lower limit of the acceptance criteria, when comparing F1 as reference formulation and F3 as test formulation, but this value is determined by the percentage of sodium alendronate dissolved in the second half of the period of the dissolution test, after t = 6 hours. In the first part of the test, especially in the first two hours, at pH 1.2, the two formulations have very different dissolution profiles.

http://dx.doi.org/10.5772/59510

3. Investigation of the influence of some absorption promoters on the release of alendronate sodium in modified release matrix tablets

Chitosan is a natural polysaccharide produced by the partial deacetylation of chitin which includes in its structure two copolymers: N-acetylglucosamine and glucosamine (Figure 3). This biodegradable and biocompatible polymer was investigated in various pharmaceutical formulations as absorption promoter, excipient for controlled release tablets or bio-mucoadhesive preparations [48].

Chitosan is soluble in acidic media, pH < 6.5, when the amino groups in its structure are protonated. At pH values > 7, the solubility of chitosan is lower, the occurrence of the transition from the solution to the gel state, which gives chitosan unique properties as an absorption promoter for the oral administration of hydrophilic macromolecular substances including peptides and proteins [49-52]. Some quaternary chitosan derivatives, for example, trimethyl chitosan (TMC), are soluble in a higher pH range (pH=1-9) in a concentration of up to 10% m/m, which results in widening the scope and applicability in this field.

The main action mechanism of CHT and TMC as absorption promoters is to open the intercellular junctions at membrane level, as a result of the interaction between CHT or its positively charged derivative and the negative charges of the sialic acid present in the intestinal mucosa. The absorption of the drug substance is therefore facilitated by para- and transcellular mechanisms [53-58].

In this study we aimed to analyze the influence of the two main absorption promoters, CHT and TMC, on the release of alendronate sodium in modified release matrix tablets based on Carbopols.

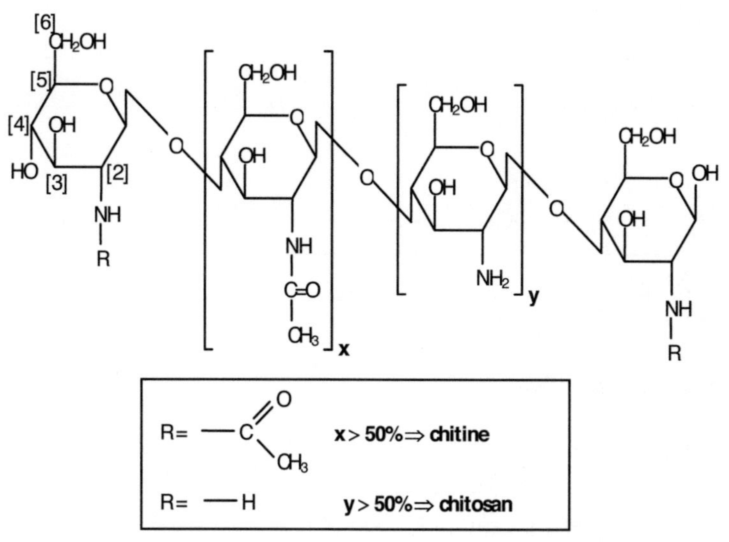

Figure 3. Chitosan - chemical structure

3.1. Materials and methods

3.1.1. Materials

Sodium alendronate trihydrate (Apotex Pharmaceutics INC, USA), *Carbopol 974 P NF, 971 P NF, 71 G NF* (Noveon Inc.), *Ludipress LCE* (BASF), *Aerosil* 200 (Degussa), *Magnesium stearate* (Union Derlivan S.A. Spain), high molecular weight *Chitosan* (CHTh) (degree of deacetylation > 85%, Aldrich), N - *Trimethyl chitosan* (G.L.S. Chemicals & Materials, India).

3.1.2. Methods

3.1.2.1. Preparation of matrix tablets

Nine alendronate sodium matrix tablets formulas were formulated and subjected to direct compression in a tablet machine Korsh EK0 (punch diameter 9 mm, 8.10 kN compression force). Table 4 presents the raw materials used in the preparation of studied formulations.

Ingredients (mg %)	Formulation								
	F1	F2	F3	F4	F5	F6	F7	F8	F9
C 71	15	–	–	15	–	–	15	–	–
C 971	–	15	15	–	15	15	–	15	15
C 974	–	–	2	–	–	2	–	–	2
CHT	–	–	–	6	6	6	–	–	–
TMC	–	–	–	–	–	–	6	6	6
AL	13.05	13.05	13.05	13.05	13.05	13.05	13.05	13.05	13.05
Mg stearate	0.5	0.5	0.8	0.5	0.5	0.8	0.5	5	0.8
Aerosil	–	0.5	1.5	–	0.5	1.5	–	5	1.5
Ludipress LCE	71.45	70.95	67.65	65.45	64.95	61.65	65.45	64.95	61.65

Table 4. Pharmaceutical formulations of modified release matrix tablets with AL-Na based on Carbopols, with absorption promoters

3.1.2.2. *"In vitro" dissolution studies*

"In vitro" dissolution tests were carried out on a *SR 8 Plus Series* (AB & L Jasco) device, under the following experimental protocol described in section I. The tests were carried out on a total of six tablets and the results shown are the average of the six determinations.

The analysis of the difference factor $f_1$and similarity factor f_2 was performed according to the equations described in Section I.

http://dx.doi.org/10.5772/59510

3.2. Results and discussions

The results of the *in vitro* dissolution test shown in Figure 4 reveal that the AL-Na release profile of the Carbopol-based matrix tablets is maintained even in the presence of CHT. It is worth noting that the released AL-Na amount for formula F5 is approximately 5% lower than for formula F2 without CHT. This result can be explained by the different behavior of CHT at the two pH values.

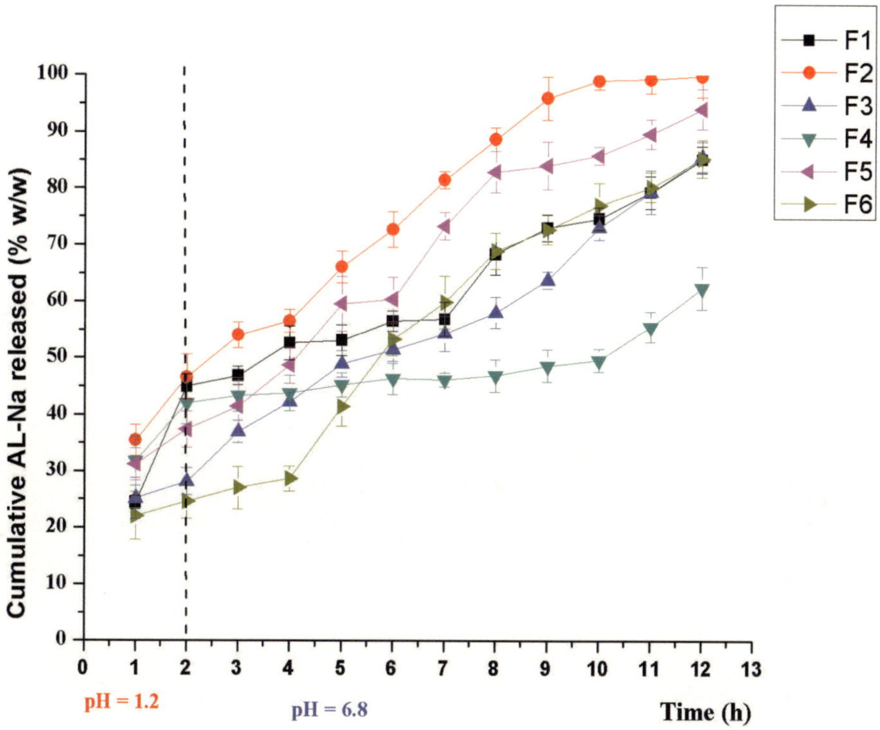

Figure 4. *In vitro* AL dissolution profile in F1-F6 formulas

To reveal the influence of CHT on the alendronate sodium release profile in modified release matrix tablets, we calculated the two control factors f_1 and f_2. The results obtained are presented in Table 5 and show that the dissolution profile is different in formulations F4 and F5 compared to formulas F1 and F2. The comparative analysis of formula F6 as test and formula F3 as reference led to a similarity factor value f_2 greater than 50 ($f_2 = 57.187$), which means that CHT does not alter the dissolution profile for this formulation. We assume that the mechanism by which CHT influences AL-Na dissolution is based on the low solubility of CHT at pH 6.8. In the case of F6, there is also the influence of C 974, which, as we noted in the previous section, due to its high crosslinking degree, causes a slower hydration of the matrix. In this context we argue that between CHT and C 974 there is a synergism of action on the release profile of alendronate sodium in modified release matrix tablets.

Reference formula (R_t)	Test formula (T_t)	f_1	f_2
F1	F4	28.991	31.947
F2	F5	12.422	46.748
F3	F6	10.799	*57.187*

Table 5. Values of f_1 and f_2 factors obtained in the comparative analysis F1-F3 versus F4-F6

The comparative results of TMC-containing formulations F7-F9 to formulations F1-F3 are shown in Figure 5.

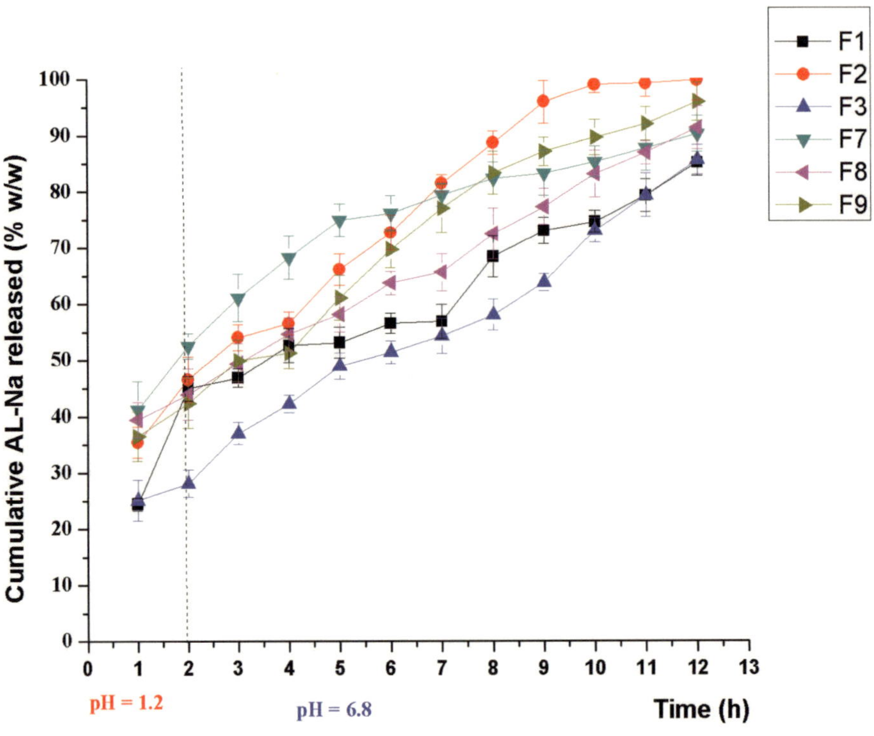

Figure 5. *In vitro* AL dissolution profile in F1-F3-F7-F9 formulas

From the analysis of the data obtained we find that all formulas in which we introduced TMC provide an alendronate sodium release in percentages above 90% during the 12 hours of the dissolution test. For this absorption promoter as well we assume that the influence on the dissolution profile of AL-Na is based on the TMC optimal solubility in the two dissolution media, a property which determined the proper hydration of the matrix tablet, thus facilitating the diffusion and release of alendronate sodium in the matrix. Difference factor f_1 and similarity factor f_2 have values that reveal for formulations F7-F9 a different release profile compared to reference formulations F1-F3 (Table 6).

http://dx.doi.org/10.5772/59510

Reference formula (R_t)	Test formula (T_t)	f_1	f_2
F1	F7	23.247	39.942
F2	F8	13.119	47.307
F3	F9	27.969	39.230

Table 6. Values of f_1 and f_2 factors obtained in the comparative analysis F1-F3 versus F7-F9

3.3. Conclusions

The comparative analysis of the results obtained from the *in vitro* dissolution test showed that formulas containing absorption promoters have an alendronate sodium dissolution profile that differs from the formulas of the modified release matrix tablets based on Carbopol without absorption promoters, test formulas (F1-F3). This conclusion is confirmed by the values of the two parameters assessing the dissolution profile: difference factor f_1 and similarity factor f_2. The influence of absorption promoters on the AL-Na dissolution profile in the studied modified release matrix tablets can be assigned to the different solubility of CHT and TMC in the two dissolution media.

4. Assessment of the release kinetics of alendronate sodium in modified-release matrix tablets

The analysis of the release kinetics of a drug substance from a dosage form is particularly important in characterizing and defining the pharmacotechnical and biopharmaceutical properties of that particular preparation. In the case of the modified release tablets based on matrix forming hydrophilic polymers, in order to determine the mechanism by which the drug is released and its evolution over time, the understanding of its kinetic release profile is a prerequisite.

The objective of this study is to identify a representative pattern for each formulation studied; taking into account the multiple formulation factors that may influence drug substance release from the modified-release matrix tablet.

4.1. Materials and methods

4.1.1. Materials

Sodium alendronate trihydrate (Apotex Pharmaceutics INC, USA), *Carbopol 974 P NF, 971 P NF, 71 G NF* (Noveon Inc.), *Ludipress LCE* (BASF), *Aerosil* 200 (Degussa), *Magnesium stearate* (Union Derlivan SA Spain), high molecular weight *chitosan* (CHTh) (degree of deacetylation > 85%, Aldrich), *N - Trimethyl chitosan* (G.L.S. Chemicals & Materials, India).

4.1.2. Methods

4.1.2.1. Preparation of matrix tablets

Nine formulations of matrix tablets with alendronate sodium were prepared by the direct compression method according to data presented in Table 4, section II.1.

4.1.2.2. "In vitro" dissolution studies

"In vitro" dissolution tests were carried out on a *SR 8 Plus Series* device, under the following experimental protocol described in section I. The tests were carried out on a total of six tablets and the results shown are the average of the six determinations.

4.1.2.3. Data fitting and kinetics of drug release

The kinetics of AL-Na release from the formulations studied was analyzed by fitting on five mathematical models according to the following equations:

The equations corresponding to the models applied in the study are:

$$\text{The zero-order kinetics:} M_t = K_0 \cdot t \tag{3}$$

$$\text{The first-order kinetics:} M_t = 100 \cdot (1 - e^{-k \cdot t}) \tag{4}$$

$$\text{Higuchi release model:} M_t = K_H \cdot t^{0.5} \tag{5}$$

$$\text{The Korsmeyer-Peppas releasemodel:} M_t = K_p \cdot t^n \quad (n = 0.45) \tag{6}$$

$$\text{The Hopfenberg release model: } M_t = 100 \cdot [1 - (1 - K_{HF} \cdot t)^n] \ (n = 2; n = 3) \tag{7}$$

where:

M_t = the amount of the drug dissolved at time t;

K_0 = zero order rate constant;

K = first order rate constant;

K_H = Higuchi rate constant;

K_P = Korsmeyer-Peppas rate constant;

K_{HF} = Hopfenberg rate constant;

n = the release exponent which characterizes the mechanism of drug release;

http://dx.doi.org/10.5772/59510

t = time

Data fitting was performed by linear and nonlinear regression, using Matlab 7.1 software.

The Akaike index (AIC) and the correlation coefficient R^2 were the criteria for the selection of the model which describes with the highest fidelity the release profile for each formulation studied. The best model prediction requires that the value of R^2 is as close as possible to 1, and the Akaike index has the smallest values [59-61].

The two model prediction parameters were calculated according to the following equations:

$$AIC = n \cdot \ln(SSR / n) + 2 \cdot p \tag{8}$$

where:

n = number of data points;

SSR = sum of squared errors;

p = number of estimated parameters.

$$R^2 = 1 - \frac{\sum_{i-1}^{n} \left((yi - y\hat{\ } i)^2 \right)}{\sum_{i-1}^{n} (yi - \bar{y})^2} \tag{9}$$

where:

y_i = data obtained experimentally;

$y\hat{\ }i$ = values approximated by the model;

$\bar{y}$ = average of experimental values

4.2. Results and discussions

The results obtained from fitting data on the five experimental models are shown in Table 7 and Figures 6-11.

Analyzing these data we can see that the zero-order release kinetic model is not representative for the formulations studied (Figure 6); this conclusion was predictable considering the data in the literature according to which this model is representative for the description of the release profile of drug substances in osmotic systems with a constant speed independent of the concentration (62-65). Mention should be made that the inclusion in the formula of C 74, a polymer with a high degree of crosslinking which causes a reduction in the rate of matrix hydration in an acidic environment, has led to good values of parameter R^2. However, the values of the Akaike index are not representative as to validate the zero-order kinetic release model for the formulations containing this polymer (Table 7).

The fitting of data from the nine formulas analyzed on the Higuchi and Korsmeyer-Peppas models confirms the release of alendronate sodium in Carbopol-based matrix tablets by a process of diffusion. The values of the parameters of the equation corresponding to the Higuchi model are representative enough to suggest that the release of the active substance in the studied matrices occurs through a diffusion process based on Fick's law according to which the release of the active substance is directly proportional to the square root of time. The Korsmeyer-Peppas model, where n is equal to 0.5 defines the active substance release through a phenomenon of Fickian diffusion from plane shapes. Fitting on this model is further substantiated by the data obtained in previous studies in which we have investigated the hydration behavior of matrix tablets, when we found an increase in direct proportion between the diameter and the thickness of the matrix, leading to the preservation of the plane geometric shape [39, 40].

Kinetic model	Parameters of model	Formulation F1	F2	F3	F4	F5	F6	F7	F8	F9
Zero-order	K_0	8.3238	10.2973	7.6325	7.9905	9.4400	7.8339	9.6863	8.8962	9.6104
	R^2	0.8401	0.9073	***0.9511***	0.8678	0.8990	***0.9678***	0.7391	0.8765	0.9036
	AIC	73.12	72.36	***59.09***	70.98	70.50	***50.12***	82.49	73.56	72.38
First-order	K	0.1900	0.2500	0.1200	0.1700	0.2100	0.1500	0.2600	0.1800	0.2100
	R^2	0.9371	***0.9758***	0.9572	0.9138	0.9677	0.9460	0.9514	0.9308	0.9624
	AIC	57.95	***43.41***	48.59	59.70	44.21	52.35	55.10	56.43	48.44
Higuchi	K_H	24.7646	30.3197	22.2784	23.7095	27.7771	22.5600	29.1919	26.4044	28.3790
	R^2	***0.9652***	***0.9885***	***0.9720***	***0.9646***	***0.9728***	***0.9391***	***0.9364***	***0.9763***	***0.9871***
	AIC	***42.33***	***32.38***	***37.67***	***41.67***	***41.41***	***54.16***	***56.61***	***40.81***	***32.29***
Korsmeyer-Peppas	K_P	27.4199	33.5240	24.6139	26.2487	30.7108	24.8812	32.3696	29.2325	31.3944
	R^2	***0.9726***	***0.9862***	***0.9631***	***0.9697***	***0.9697***	***0.9214***	***0.9565***	***0.9814***	***0.9872***
	AIC	***37.12***	***36.96***	***42.47***	***37.41***	***43.82***	***57.80***	***50.42***	***34.65***	***30.73***
Hopfenberg (n=2)	K_{HF}	0.0548	0.0844	0.0495	0.0521	0.0679	0.0517	0.0686	0.0612	0.0703
	R^2	0.9160	0.9835	0.9631	0.9228	0.9575	0.9806	0.08664	0.9499	0.9771
	AIC	65.57	47.84	50.97	64.66	54.60	41.43	73.27	65.06	58.29
Hopfenberg (n=3)	K_{HF}	0.0405	0.0706	0.0363	0.0383	0.0521	0.0382	0.0522	0.0461	0.0545
	R^2	0.9324	*0.9732*	*0.9562*	0.9290	*0.9672*	*0.9794*	0.9022	0.9578	0.9840
	AIC	62.95	*44.36*	*48.73*	62.55	*49.26*	*42.77*	70.05	62.21	53.58

Table 7. Parameter values of the mathematical equations corresponding to the evaluation models of release kinetics and their predictability indicators

Data fitting on the Hopfenberg model revealed the presence and involvement of the erosion phenomenon in the process of release of alendronate sodium. The prediction parameter R^2 has acceptable values (> 0.90) for all formulations studied, but the Akaike index does not allow the validation of this model, regardless of the value of n. According to data obtained from the analysis of the hydration behavior of matrices, erosion increases after 7-8 hours after the introduction of the matrix in the dissolution medium. Figures 10-11 show a good fitting of the model particularly for formulations based on C 971, C 971 associated with C 974, as well as in similar formulas in which we introduced CHT and TMC after moment 6-7 of the study. Therefore, we consider that the Akaike index values are determined by the nonlinearity of the erosion process.

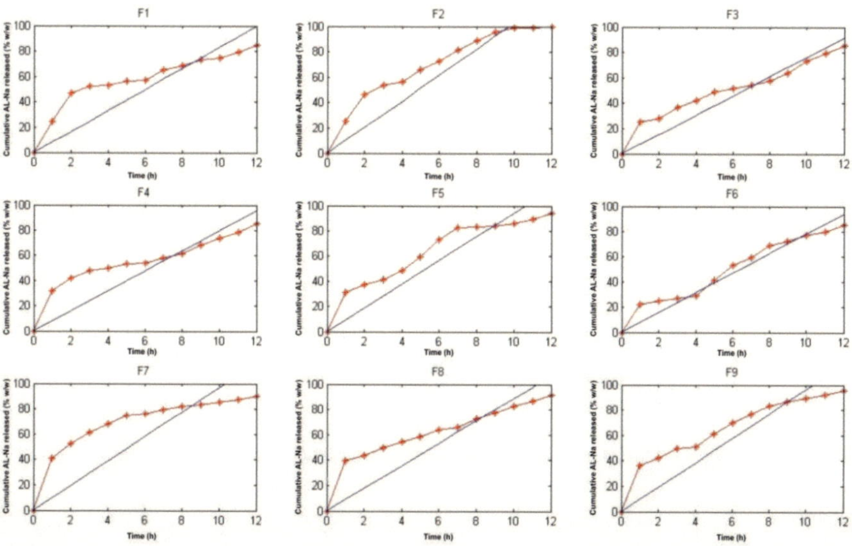

Figure 6. The fitting plot of the AL-Na dissolution profiles from formulations F1-F9 with the zero-order kinetics model

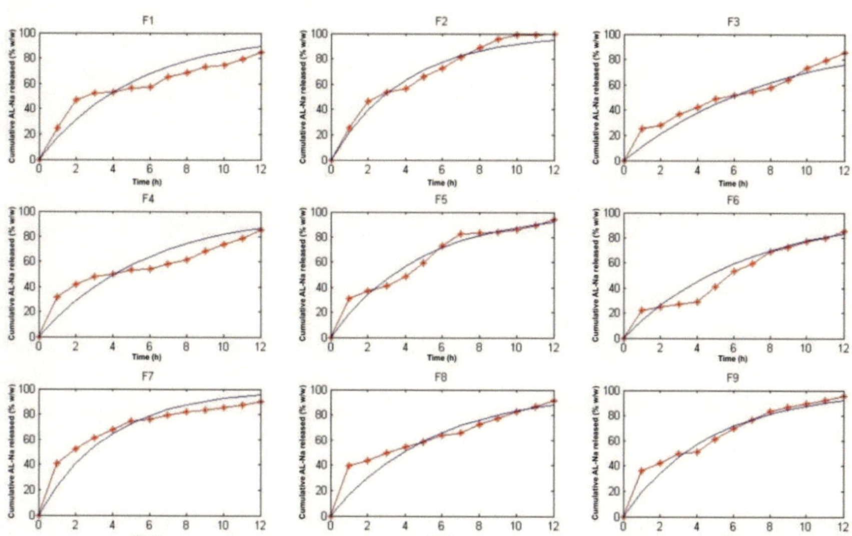

Figure 7. The fitting plot of the AL-Na dissolution profiles from formulations F1-F9 with the first-order kinetics model

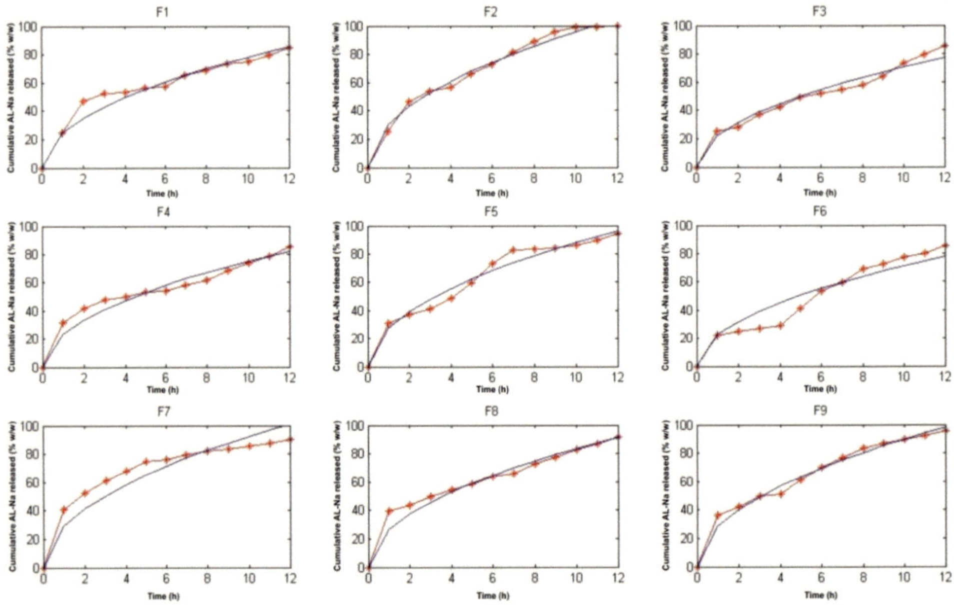

Figure 8. The fitting plot of the AL-Na dissolution profiles from formulations F1-F9 with the Higuchi model

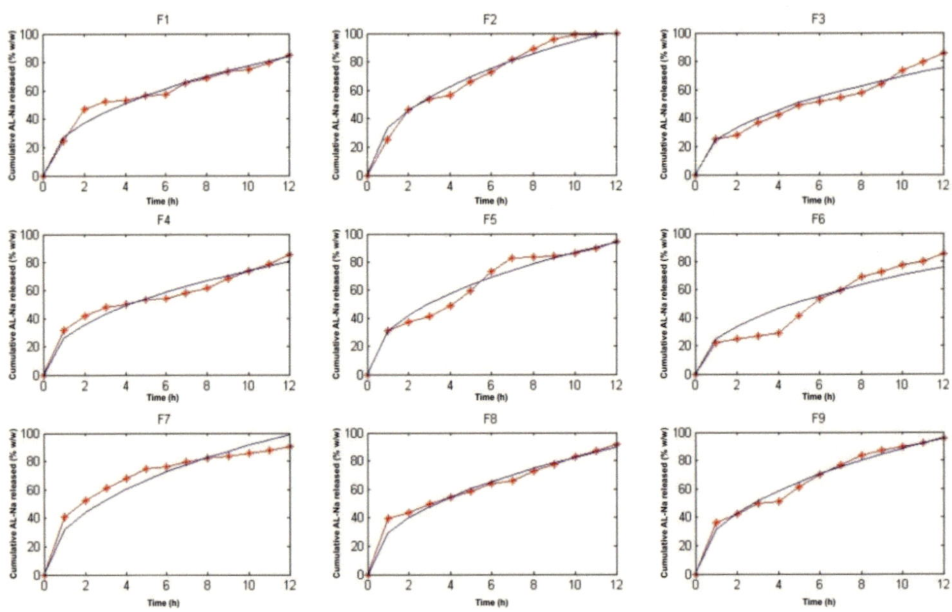

Figure 9. The fitting plot of the AL-Na dissolution profiles from formulations F1-F9 with the Korsmeyer-Peppas model

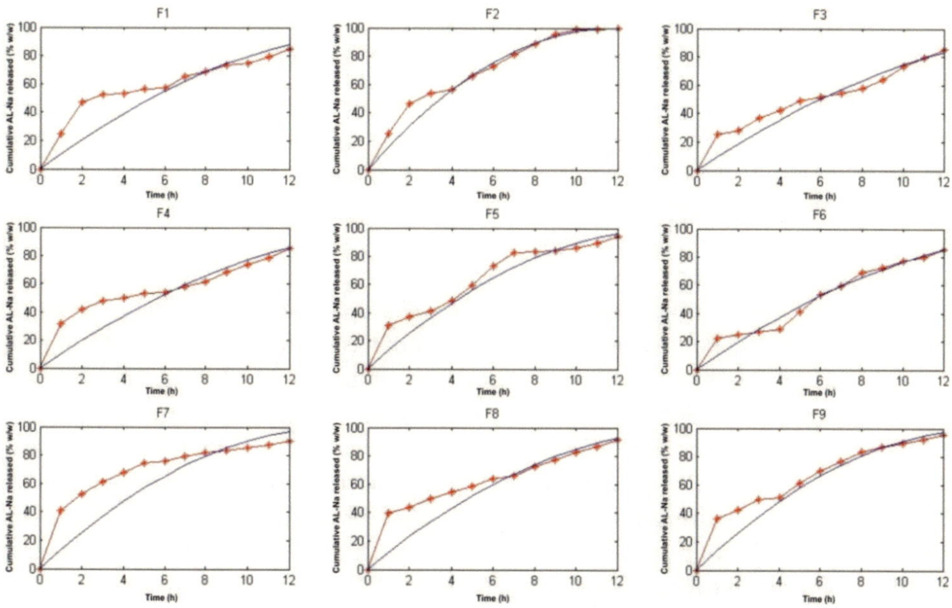

Figure 10. The fitting plot of the AL-Na dissolution profiles from formulations F1-F9 with the Hopfenberg (n=2) model

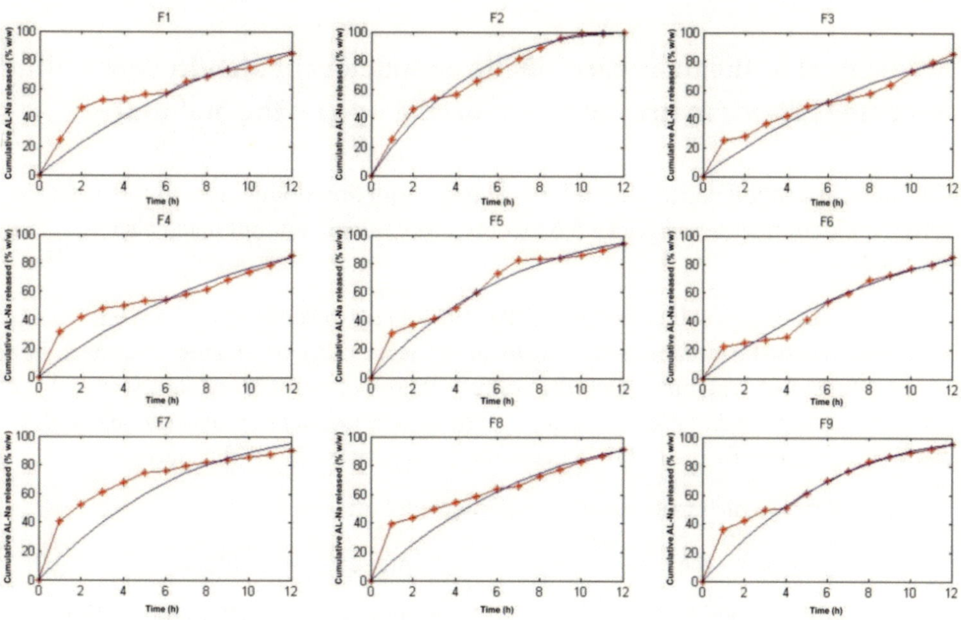

Figure 11. The fitting plot of the AL-Na dissolution profiles from formulations F1-F9 with the Hopfenberg model (n=3)

4.3. Conclusions

The results obtained showed good data fitting on the Higuchi model for all formulations studied, which leads to the conclusion that AL-Na release from hydrophilic matrix tablets occurs through a diffusion process based on Fick's law. In addition, the results obtained when fitting data on the Korsmeyer-Peppas mathematical model is an additional argument for considering diffusion as the main mechanism of AL-Na release from flat modified-release hydrophilic matrix tablets. The Hopfenberg model applied to modified-release matrix tablets with a complex formulation based on combinations of matrix-forming polymers in order to highlight the involvement of erosion in the process of active substance release generated a good fitting of the data in the analysis of the correlation coefficient R^2, but the Akaike index has high values, which does not allow the validation of the model. Data analysis shows that in the second half of the duration of the dissolution test, the data obtained experimentally generate a better fitting for the Hopfenberg model both for $n = 2$ and for $n = 3$. In conclusion, the data obtained from fitting on the Hopfenberg model confirms the involvement of erosion as a mechanism of alendronate sodium release from modified-release hydrophilic matrix tablets, but the predictive parameter values of the model do not allow the validation of this model due to the nonlinearity of erosion.

In conclusion, Fickian diffusion is the main mechanism of alendronate sodium release from modified-release hydrophilic matrix tablets and erosion is the secondary mechanism.

5. Assessment of the pharmacokinetic parameters of alendronate sodium in modified-release matrix tablets administered on the oral route

Alendronate absorption occurs through passive diffusion, predominantly in the upper small intestine (duodenum, jejunum, pH = 6-6.5), only a very small amount being also absorbed at the gastric level [66].

Alendronate has a low oral bioavailability (0.6 to 0.9%) for doses ranging from 5 to 70 mg, in conventional release formulations administered in the morning on an empty stomach or two hours after breakfast. The bioavailability of the 10 mg tablet is 0.59, while the weekly dose administration of 70 mg in tablets or solution leads to a bioavailability of 0.64% [67, 68]. These values are determined by the following general characteristics of bisphosphonates:

- low lipophilicity, which restricts intra-and intercellular transport;
- high polarity given by the negative charge, which prevents paracellular transport [69].

Plasma *distribution* of alendronate exhibits very low concentrations (<5 ng/ml) at therapeutic doses. Plasmatic $t_{1/2}$ of alendronate is short 0.5 to 2 h compared to $t_{1/2}$ in deposits at the site of bone resorption that have values expressed in years for alendronate being > 10 years. Alendronate binds to plasma proteins in the ratio of 78% and also forms complexes with some divalent cations, eg calcium, magnesium, iron [70].

Excretion of alendronate is in the ratio of 99% in the feces and only 0.4% of the amount absorbed is eliminated through the kidneys by glomerular filtration and tubular excretion.

Storage of alendronate in the bone tissue depends on the affinity for hydroxyapatite, the *in vitro* affinity constant $K_{L\ alendronat}$ 2.9 x 10^6 mol/l [71].

Pharmacokinetically, alendronate does not present any significant differences between the main groups of patients. The oral bioavailability of this active substance is similar in both children and adults [66, 72]. The main objective of these studies is to evaluate the pharmacokinetic parameters of alendronate administered as modified-release matrix tablets.

5.1. Materials and methods

5.1.1. Materials

According to the results obtained in the research presented in subsections I-III, in order to achieve the pharmacokinetic studies we selected matrix tablets formulas that exhibited optimal characteristics of release (Table 8).

Ingredients (mg %)	Formulation			
	F2	F5	F8	Fm
C 971	15	15	15	-
CHTh	-	6	-	-
TMC	-	-	6	-
AL	13.05	13.05	13.05	13.05
Mg Stearate	0.5	0.5	0.5	0.5
Aerosil	0.5	0.5	0.5	0.5
Ludipress LCE	70.95	64.95	64.95	85.95

Table 8. The formulations of modified-release matrix tablets containing alendronate sodium

The tablets used in pharmacological research were prepared by direct compression, in accordance with the technology described in Section I.

5.1.2. Methods

5.1.2.1. Experimental protocol

The research was performed on adult male dogs weighing 30-40 kg, divided into four groups of 2 animals. Samples containing 20 mg alendronate sodium/tablet corresponding to the three formulations studied were denoted F2, F5, F8. Fm, the control sample, comprised immediate-release tablets with Alendronate sodium. The samples were administered to the four groups as follows:

- F2 → group I;
- F5 → group II;
- F8 → group III
- Fm → group IV.

The experimental study was conducted over a period of 48 hours and the tablets were administered orally after the animals had fasted for 12 hours. During the experiment, the animals had free access to water and food, except for 4 hours of food deprivation following the administration of tablets.

Mention should be made that in the literature we did not identify the lethal dose 50 (DL 50) of alendronate sodium administered to dogs, being conducted research by administering 200 mg / kg, a dose for which a mild renal toxicity was recorded [8, 73].

Preparation of the animals: 7 days prior to the experiment, each animal had free access to food and water and was kept under normal conditions of light and temperature.

Blood sampling was performed using the following procedure:

- in order to collect the blood samples a catheter was placed in the femoral vein;
- to characterize the pharmacokinetic parameters, samples of 4 ml of blood were collected at each moment in heparin vacutainers;
- sampling times were as follows: M 0 - prior to administration; M 1 - 30 min. after administration; M 2 - 1 h after administration; M 3 - 1 h and 30 min. after administration; M 4 - 2 hours after administration; M 5 - 2 h and 30 min. after administration; M 6 - 3 hours after administration; M 7 - 3 h and 30 min. after administration; M 8 - 4 hours after administration; M 9 - 6 hours after administration; M 10 - 8 h after administration; M 11 - 10 h after administration; M 12 - 12 h after administration; M 13 - 24 hours after administration;

Processing of the blood samples consisted in:

- centrifugation after 30 minutes from collecting, at a speed of 3000 rpm, for 10 min.;
- serum was transferred into Ependorff test tubes and stored in a freezer, at – 20 °C, until the HPLC quantitative analysis, according to the method described in section I.

All animals used in this study were clinically healthy and haematological and biochemical analyses had been performed prior to the experiment.

5.1.2.2. Calculation of pharmacokinetic parameters

The main pharmacokinetic parameters that were evaluated directly, without a pharmacokinetic modeling, based on the experimental data, are: *the coordinates of the peak (C_{max} and T_{max}), the areas under the curve (AUC_{0-t}, $AUC_{0-\infty}$, $AUC_{t-\infty}$), the total clearance (Cl) and the average residual time (MRT).* These parameters are independent of the representation model of drug kinetics in the body, and are very useful in bioavailability studies. A series of other parameters depend on the pharmacokinetic model, so that it should be taken into account in calculating them.

http://dx.doi.org/10.5772/59510

In the case of extravascular administration, the following parameters dependent on the model can be calculated: *elimination rate constant* (k_e), *biological half-life* ($t_{1/2}$), *absorption rate constant* (k_a) and *volume of distribution* (V_d).

The main pharmacokinetic parameters calculated were:

- *coordinates of the peak* (C_{max} and T_{max}) – individual C_{max} values expressed in μg/ml and T_{max}, expressed in hours, were obtained from the examination of experimental data;

- *areas under the curve* (AUC_{0-t}, $AUC_{0-\infty}$, $AUC_{t-\infty}$) - the area under the plasma concentration curve, noted AUC, is a parameter that reflects the extent of absorption in the administered dose and that is proportional to the amount of drug that reaches the blood after oral administration. As a result, this parameter is essential for the determination of bioavailability.

- the *area under the experimental plasmatic concentration curve* AUC_{0-t} was calculated by using the trapezoidal rule, which is the most common method. We calculated the area from time zero (initial time) to the time when the last blood sample was collected to determine the concentration of the drug substance. The area under the curve is equal to the sum of the areas of the trapezoids realized between two concentrations corresponding to two successive collections of blood samples. The area of each trapezoid was calculated according to the equation:

$$S_i = \frac{c_i + c_{i+1}}{2}(t_{i+1} - t_i) \tag{10}$$

Consequently,

$$AUC_0^t = \sum_{i-0}^{n-1} S_i = \sum_{i-0}^{n-1} \frac{c_i + c_{i+1}}{2}(t_{i+1} - t_i) \tag{11}$$

where, n = number of trapezoids in which we divide the area under the curve (n is the number of collections of biological samples);

- the *total area under the plasmatic concentration curve* $AUC_{0-\infty}$ is equal to the sum of the area under the experimental concentration curve and the area extrapolated from the time of the last sample collection to infinity.

$AUC_{0-\infty}$ was calculated using the equation:

$$AUC_0^\infty = AUC_0^t + AUC_t^\infty = \sum_{i-0}^{n-1} \frac{c_i + c_{i+1}}{2}(t_{i+1} - t_i) + \frac{c_n}{k_e}, \tag{12}$$

where ke is calculated based on the end points of the plasma concentration curve in time.

- the *extrapolated area* is the area from the last sampling time extrapolated to infinity and it was calculated by the equation:

$$AUC_t^{\infty} = \frac{c_n}{k_e} \tag{13}$$

where cn is plasma concentration of the last determination.

Totalclearance (Cl) – for oral administration, the absorbed dose and the total clearance cannot be calculated exactly, so we determined the ratio:

$$\frac{Cl}{F} = \frac{dose}{AUC} \tag{14}$$

where F – correction factor

- the *elimination rate constant (k_e)* was determined by the method of residuals, based on plasmatic concentrations of the drug substance determined at different time intervals. This method is also called the "least squares method" or the "method of the least sums of the squares errors" and is used to estimate the true values with the help of the experimentally determined values.
- *biological half-life ($t_{1/2}$)* was calculated by the mathematical method. Starting from the equation of the plasma concentration dependent on time in the disposal phase

$$c(t) = C_0 e^{-k_e t} \tag{15}$$

and knowing that the initial concentration is Co, and at the time t1/2 concentration is reduced by half, the equation becomes

$$C_0 = \frac{C_0}{2} e^{-k_e t_{1/2}} \tag{16}$$

from which we obtain:

$$t_{1/2} = \frac{\ln C_0 - \ln \frac{C_0}{2}}{k_e} = \frac{\ln 2}{k_e} = \frac{0.693}{k_e} \tag{17}$$

where: k_e was obtained by linear regression as a slope of the terminal phase of the logarithmically transformed plasma concentration curve versus time

http://dx.doi.org/10.5772/59510

- *volume of distribution* (V_d) – similar to total clearance, V_d cannot be evaluated exactly for extravascular administration. Therefore the ratio is calculated:

$$\frac{V}{F} = \frac{dose}{k_e \cdot AUC_0^{\infty}} \tag{18}$$

Statistical analysis of data was performed using the PHARM-STAT program for the investigation of bioavailability.

5.2. Results and discussion

5.2.1. Bioavailability of alendronate sodium in modified-release hydrophilic matrix tablets based on Carbopol

Results from the comparative analysis of serum concentrations of alendronate administered as immediate-release tablets to the animals in (control) group IV and as modified-release matrix tablets to group I, show a higher absorption of alendronate sodium from the modified-release tablets.

We can distinguish two major phases in the evolution of the absorption of alendronate, in close correlation with the swelling characteristics of matrix tablets. Modified-release matrix tablets with sodium alendronate administered to the animals in group I generate an absorption maximum at 2.5 to 3 hours, after which there is a plateau condition in the concentration range of 0.25 to 0.30 μg/mL alendronate until time 12, i.e. 10 hours after administration (Figure 12).

Initially, in the first 1.5 hours after administration, the animals in control group IV exhibit an alendronate serum concentration that is higher compared to group I. Subsequently, after about 2 hours from the administration, when the matrix tablet has hydrated and the phenomenon of alendronate diffusion in the inner matrix layers occurs, the serum concentration of alendronate in the animals in group I increases significantly (Figure 13)

By analyzing the data obtained, we consider that the formulation of alendronate in matrix tablets based on Carbopol C 971 resulted in a considerable increase in oral bioavailability.

5.2.2. Bioavailability of alendronate sodium in modified-release hydrophilic matrix tablets in the presence of absorption promoters

In the first hour after administration, the animals in the control group had a higher serum concentration of alendronate compared to the modified-release formulations (Figure 14). Subsequently, at collection time 4, that is 1.5 hours after administration, the formulation corresponding to the modified-release matrix tablets containing trimethil chitosan as an absorption promoter exhibits the highest concentration. This superiority lasts until time 5, that is 3 hours after administration (Figure 15). According to these results, we consider that over this time the absorption enhancer action of trimethilchitosan manifests itself.

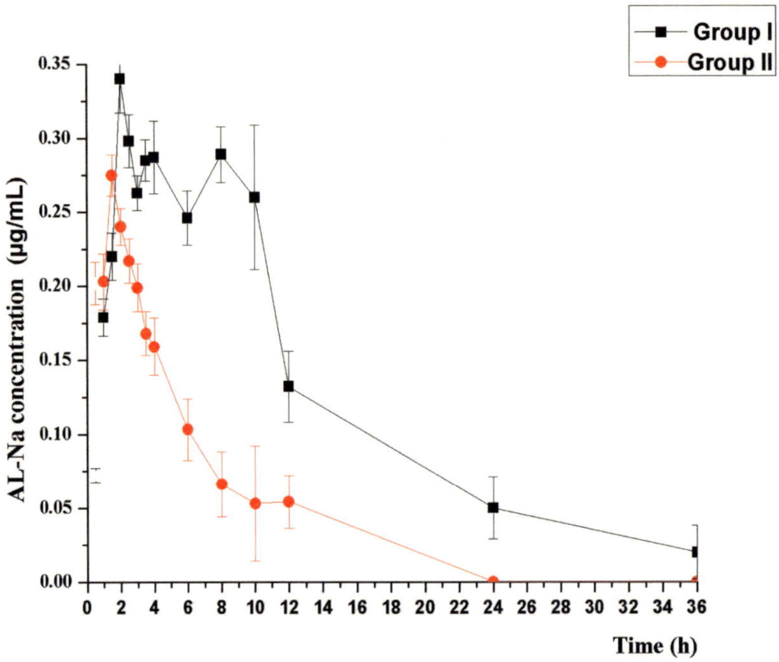

Figure 12. *In vivo* release of AL-Na from hydrophilic matrix tablets with modified release (0-12 hours)

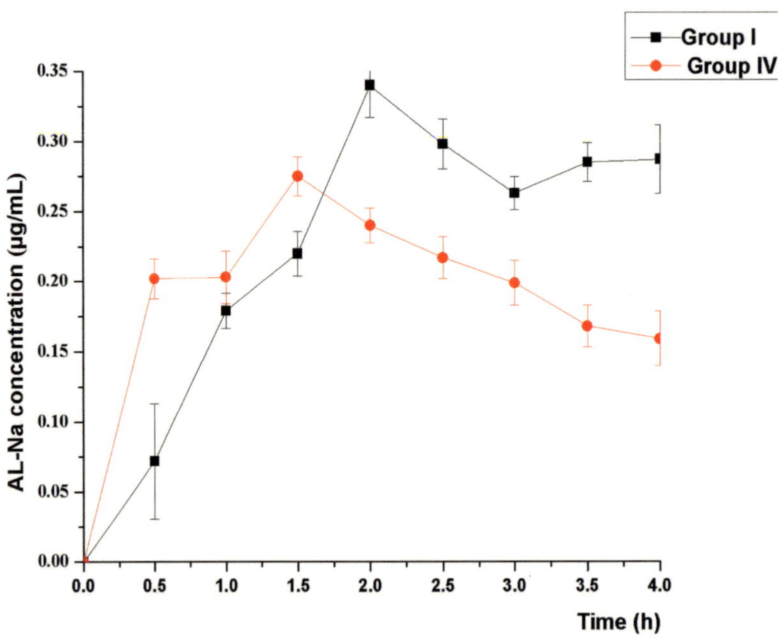

Figure 13. *In vivo* release of AL-Na from hydrophilic matrix tablets with modified release (0-4 hours)

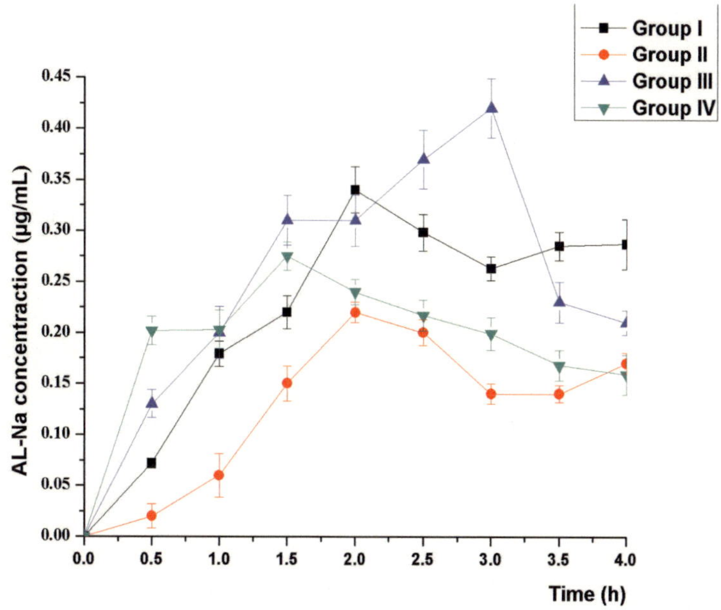

Figure 14. In vivo release of AL-Na from hydrophilic matrix tablets with modified release in the presence of absorption promotors (0-4 hours)

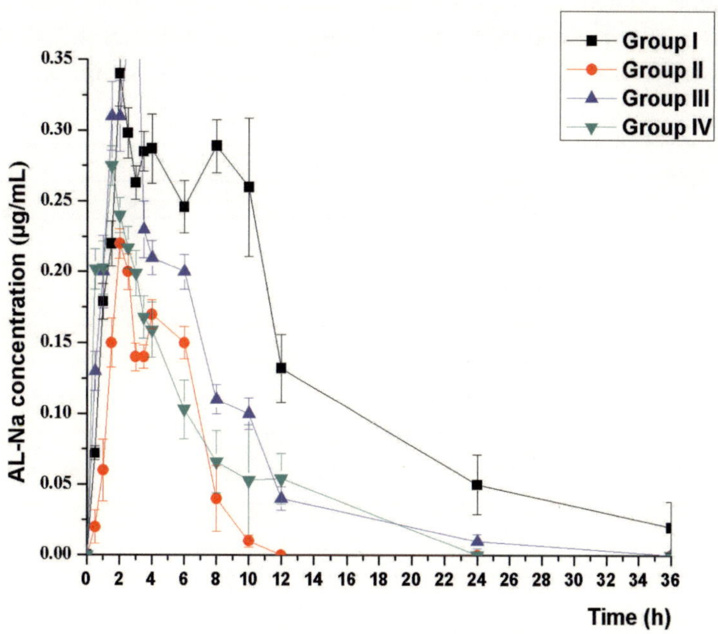

Figure 15. In vivo release of alendronate sodium from hydrophilic matrix tablets with modified release (0-12 hours)

An unexpected development was recorded for animals in group II, which were administered modified-release matrix tablets in which we had introduced chitosan as an absorption promoter. The serum concentration of alendronate in this group was lower than in the control formula throughout the experiment. There are two surprising aspects related to this: on the one hand, the fact that chitosan does not act as absorption promoter and, on the other, that there occurs a cancellation of the retardation effect and of the release optimization resulting from the administration of the modified-release of matrix tablets based on Carbopol.

5.2.3. Pharmacokinetic parameters: Cmax, Tmax, $t_{1/2}$, areas under the curve

The comprehensive review of the individual values of plasma concentrations over time and of the corresponding individual graphs allows for a primary pharmacokinetic analysis of results. Based on plasma concentration values over time the pharmacokinetic parameters (T_{max}, C_{max}, $AUC_{0\text{-}t}$, $AUC_{0\text{-}\infty}$, $AUC_{t\text{-}\infty}$, Cl, k_e, $t_{1/2}$, V_d) were determined. Subsequently, the data were analyzed statistically to determine the possible existence of significant differences.

Mean C_{max} peak plasma concentrations (Table 9) of the modified-release matrix tablets and of the formula related to the control group, respectively, in a single dose study, reveal differences between the formulations studied. Thus, for formula F2 given to group I, C_{max} = 0,34μg/ml, formula F5 associated with group II provides a C_{max} = 0.24 μg/ml, formula F8, group III, has C_{max} = 0.48 μg/ml, and the control formula given to group IV, C_{max} = 0.28 μg/ml. Result processing through the ANOVA test shows that the differences between peak plasma concentrations after administration of formulation F2, compared to control formulation and after administration of F8 compared to the control, are not statistically significant. For parameter Cmax only the differences between group I and III are statistically significant.

Mean value	GROUP			
	I	II	III	IV
C_{max}	0.34	0.24	0.48	0.28
T_{max}	2.00	2.25	3.00	1.50
$AUC_{0\text{-}t}$	2.93	1.28	2.65	1.94
$AUC_{0\text{-}\infty}$	3.17	1.40	2.72	1.94
$AUC_{t\text{-}\infty}$	0.24	0.12	0.07	0.00
% AUC_{extra}	7.57	8.56	2.37	0.00
Cl	0.03	0.05	0.04	0.05
k_e	0.08	0.08	0.13	0.08
$t_{1/2}$	8.31	8.26	5.79	8.63
V_d	0.37	0.62	0.32	0.63

Table 9. Pharmacokinetic parameters of AL-Na

The mean values of time taken to reach peak concentration, T_{max} (Table 9) exhibits equal values for groups I and II compared to control group IV. The highest value was determined for group

III, i.e. T_{max} = 3 h. By applying a non-parametric test it was found that the differences are not statistically significant.

The mean of the values of the extrapolated area AUC $_{t-\infty}$ is below 20% in all situations, which proves the right choice for the last sample collection time. Analysis of the mean total area under the plasma concentration-time ($AUC_{0-\infty}$) reveals differences between products. The highest value was recorded for group I. Analysis of the mean values of Cl and V_d does not reveal statistically significant differences between products.

5.3. Conclusions

The results obtained reveal an optimization of the bioavailability of alendronate administered in modified-release matrix tablets from collection moment 5, i.e. two hours after administration, as the animals in group I, corresponding to this formula, had a serum concentration of alendronate superior to the control group.

The two absorption promoters used, trimethyl chitosan and chitosan, had completely different influences on the absorption of alendronate in the modified-release matrix tablets. Thus, trimethyl chitosan acted as an absorption promoter in the range 1.5 to 3 hours after administration, and caused the highest serum concentrations of alendronate, sometimes double compared to the control. After that moment, concentrations are above the values of the control group, but slightly lower than the values of group I, coresponding to the modified-release matrix tablets based on Carbopol.

The administration of modified release tablets with alendronate sodium in which we associated chitosan as absorption promoter has led to surprising results, because over the whole experiment, the serum concentration of alendronate sodium was lower than of group IV (control group). Chitosan exhibited virtually no absorption promoting action; it additionally canceled the release retardation and optimization effect proved on group I after the administration of alendronate in modified-release matrix tablets based on carbopol.

6. Conclusions

The crosslinking degree of Carbopol has a major influence on the release properties of the hydrophilic matrix tablets. The C71 and C971 Carbopol types, having a low crosslinking degree, hydrate much better in pH 1.2, and this facilitates the AL-Na dissolution, its diffusion through the gel layers of the matrix and, consequently, an optimized release of AL-Na. On the contrary, C 971 – a polymer with a high crosslinking degree, slows the hydration process of the matrix. Sort Carbopol 71 in a concentration of 15% results in hydrophilic matrix tablets with optimal release of AL-Na. The different dissolution profile of Al-Na in the Carbopol-based modified release matrix tablets is also confirmed by the values of the two control parameters f_1 and f_2. Fitting the release data to the kinetic analysis with the Higuchi and the Korsmeyer-Peppas model confirms the release of the Al-Na in the Carbopol-based matrix tablets by a diffusion process. The Hopfenberg model applied to modified-release matrix tablets with a complex formulation based on associations of matrix-forming polymers to highlight the involvement of erosion in the release of the active substance generated a good fitting of the data ($R^2 > 0.90$), but the high values of the Akaike index do not allow the validation of the model. *In vivo* studies have shown a higher bioavailability of AL-Na in modified release matrix tablets at 1.5 hours after dosing. The results of the evaluation of the *in vivo* AL-Na release indicate the optimization of the bioavailability of AL-Na in the Carbopol 71-based matrix tablets, the optimal concentration being reached after 2 hours from the administration of the tablet. The two absorption promoters used - chitosan and trimethyl chitosan - had a totally different effect on alendronate absorption. Trimethyl chitosan showed a strong absorption promoting effect by doubling AL-Na serum concentration while CHT did not show this effect. According to the results obtained, Carbopol 71 is a good forming agent for modified-release tablets to improve the oral bioavailability of AL-Na.

Acknowledgements

The authors express their deep gratitude to *Professor Iuliana Popovici PhD* at Grigore T. Popa University of Medicine and Pharmacy, Iasi, Romania, for her professional guidance and valuable support for this work. Our thanks also go to *Associate Professor Ileana Oana Macari PhD* at Alexandru Ioan Cuza University, Iasi, Romania, for the revision of the English version of this article.

Author details

Lacramioara Ochiuz[1*], Anca Giorgiana Grigoras[2] and Cristina Mihaela Ghiciuc[3]

*Address all correspondence to: ochiuzd@yahoo.com

1 Department of Pharmaceutical Technology, Faculty of Pharmacy, University of Medicine and Pharmacy "Grigore T. Popa", Iasi, Romania

2 "Petru Poni" Institute of Macromolecular Chemistry, Iasi, Romania

3 Faculty of Medicine, University of Medicine and Pharmacy "Grigore T. Popa", Iasi, Romania

References

[1] Whitaker M., Guo J., Kihoe T., Benson G. Bisphosphonates for osteoporosis e where do we go from here? N Engl J Med 2012;366(22):2048-51.

[2] Black D.M., Bauer D.C., Schwartz A.V., et al. Continuing bisphosphonate treatment for osteoporosis for whom and for how long? N Engl J Med 2012;366(22):2051-3.

[3] Schwartz A.V., Bauer D.C., Cummings S.R., et al. Efficacy of continued alendronate for fractures in women with and without prevalent vertebral fracture: the FLEX trial. J Bone Miner Res 2010;25:976-82.

[4] Bone H.G., Hosking D., Devogelaer J.P., et al. Ten years' experience with alendronate for osteoporosis in postmenopausal women. N Engl J Med 2004;350:1189-99.

[5] Medication Guide Fosama Plus® Reference ID: 3403221 accessed via the internet at: http://www.fda.gov/downloads/Drugs/DrugSafety (accessed 13 October 2014).

[6] Bischoff -Ferrari H.A. Optimal serum 25-hydroxyvitamin D levels for multiple health outcomes. Adv Exp Med Biol. 2008; 624: 55-71

[7] Bonnick S., Saag K., Kiel D. et al. Comparison of weekly treatment of postmenopausal osteoporosis with alendronate versus risedronate over two years. J Clin Endocrinol Metab, 2006;91, 2631-2637.

[8] Doc. Ref.: EMEA/360723/2009, accessed via the internet at http://www.emea. europa.eu/humandocs/PDFs/EPAR/Fosavance/23778305en (accessed 20 February 2013).

[9] Zarowitz B.J. Bisphosphonate Duration of Therapy for Management of Osteoporosis. J Geri Nurse 2012;33(6): 479-481.

[10] Flashner-Barak M., Rosenberg V., Dahan M., Lerner Y. Composition and dosage form for delayed gastric release of alendronate and&or other bisphosphonates, accessed vie the internet at: http://www.freepatentsonline.com/6476006 (accessed 3 March 2012).

[11] US Patent 5431920 – Enteric coated oral compositions containing bisphosphonic acid antihypercalcemic agents, accessed via the internet at: http://www.patentstorm.us/patents/5431920 (accessed 28 December 2013).

[12] Effervescent alendronate formulation, United States Patent 5853759, accessed via the internet at. http://www.freepatentsonline.com/5853759 (accessed 3 February 2014).

[13] Hodges L., Connolly S.M., Band J. et al., Gastroprotective Effects Of Effervescent Alendronate Formulation Shown By Scintigraphic and Gastric pH Monitoring, Gastroenterology, 2000;119, 631-639.

[14] Oral liquid alendronate formulations United States Patent 5462932, accessed via the internet at: http://www.freepatentsonline.com/5462932 (accessed 3 February 2014).

[15] Fulya K., Nevin, C. Development of an oral microemulsion fromulation of alendronate: effects of oil and co-surfactant type on phase behaviour, J. of Microencapsulation., 2008;5(25), 315-323.

[16] Cruz L., Assumpcao E., Guterres S. High encapsulation efficiency of sodium alendronate in Eudragit S100/HPMC blend microparticles, Quim. Nova, 2009;5(32), 1170-1174.

[17] The dispersible alendronate microparticle formulation, European Patent EP1617826, accessed via the internet at: http://www.freepatentsonline.com/EP1617826 (accessed 3 February 2014).

[18] Soula G., Guimberteau F., Castan C., Meyrueix R., Dargelas F. Microparticles With Modified Release of At Least One Active Principle and Oral Pharmaceutical Form, accessed via the internet at: http://www.faqs.org/ patents/app/20090220611 (accessed 3 February 2014)

[19] Reddy G., Kumar T., Veena K.M. Formulation and evaluation of alendronate sodium gel for the treatment of bone resorbtive lesions in periodontitis, Drug Delivery, 2005;4(12), 217-222.

[20] Vaginal delivery of bisphosphonates, US Patent 6572874, accessed via the internet at: http://www.patentstorm.us/patents/6572874 (accessed 3 February 2014).

[21] Steven C., Karen E. Intranasal delivery of the bisphosphonate alendronate in the rat and dog, Pharm. Researc, 1993;6(10), 924-933.

[22] Plaster composition comprising alendronate as an effective ingredient for treating osteoporosis, US Patent 072869, accessed via the internet at: http://www.patentstorm.us/ patents/072869 (accessed 20 February 2013).

[23] Ahyoung C., Hyesil G., Inkoo C., Hyesun G. The effects of fatty acids in propylene glycol on the percutaneous absorption of alendronate across the excited hairless skin, Int. J. Pharm., 2008;357, 126-131.

[24] Choulis N., Papadopoulis H. Timed Release Tablets Containing Quinine Sulfate, J. Pharm. Sci., 1975;64(6), 1033-1035.

[25] Seham A.E. Interaction of Verapamil Hydrochloride with Carbopol 934P and Its Effect on the Release Rate of the Drug and the Water Uptake of the Polymer Matrix, Drug Develop and Ind Pharm, 2001;27(9), 925-934.

[26] Srikonda V.S., Indra K., Khan M. Atenolol gastrointestinal therapeutic system: optimization of formulation variables using response surface methodology, J Control Release, 1997;45(2), 121-130.

[27] Singh B., Chakkal S.K., Ahuja N. Formulation and Optimization of Controlled Release Mucoadhesive Tablets of Atenolol Using Response Surface Methodology, AAPS PharmSciTech, 2006;7(1), 1208-1218.

[28] Silva M., Gurruchaga N., Goñi I. Physical blends of starch graft copolymers as matrices for colon targeting drug delivery systems, Carbohydrate Polymers, 2009;76, 593-601.

[29] Anuradha A., Pradeep R.V. Bioadhesive Ranitidine Hydrochloride for Gastroretention with Controlled Microenvironmental pH, Drug Develop and Ind Pharm, 2008;34(8), 860-869.

[30] BelgamwarV., Shah V., Surana S.J. Formulation and evaluation of oral mucoadhesive multiparticulate system containing metoprolol tartarate: an *in vitro-ex vivo* characterization, Current drug delivery., 2009;6(1), 113-121.

[31] Lubrizol Pharmaceutical Bulletin 1: "Polymers for Pharmaceutical Applications", accessed via the internet at: www.pharma.lubrizol.com (accessed 13 April 2012).

[32] Pharmaceutical Bulletin 30, Lubrizol Pharmaceutical Polymers for Controlled Release Tablets and Capsules, accessed via the internet at: www.pharma.lubrizol.com (accessed 13 April 2012).

[33] Pharmaceutical Bulletin 31, Formulating Controlled Release Tablets and Capsules with Carbopol® Polymers, accessed via the internet at: www.pharma.lubrizol.com (accessed 13 April 2012).

[34] Pharmaceutical Bulletin 32, Application of Carbopol® 71G NF Polymer in Controlled Release Tablets, accessed via the internet at: www.pharma.lubrizol.com (accessed 13 April 2012).

[35] Maderuelo C., Zarzuelo A., Lanao JM. Critical factors in the release of drugs from sustained release hydrophilic matrices. J Control Release 2011;154: 2-19.

[36] Lamberti G, Galdi I, Barba A.A. Controlled release from hydrogel-based solid matrices. A model accounting for water up-take, swelling and erosion. Int J Pharm 2011;407: 78-86.

[37] Shao Y, Li L, Gu X, Wang L, Mao S, Evaluation of chitosan-anionic polymers based tablets for extended-release of highly water soluble drugs, Asian Journal of Pharmaceutical Sciences (2014), doi: 10.1016/j.ajps.2014.08.002.

[38] Popovici I., Ochiuz L., Popa E., Dorneanu V., Saramet G., Lupuleasa D.: „Influence Of Carbomer Type On The Benzydamine Mucoadhesive Oral Tablets Formulation", European Journal of Drug Methabolism and Pharmacokinetics, vol. 32, 2007, p.89.

[39] Ochiuz L., Popa G., Gafitanu E. "Development of Hydrophilic Swellable Carbopol Matrixes for Extended Release of Alendronate Tablets", Farmacia, vol. LVI, nr. 5, 2008, p.521-531.

[40] Ochiuz L., Moscalu M., Ciobanu G. Study on the influence of formulation parameters on the pharmacotechnical characteristics of hydrophylic carbopol matrix tablets using a D-optimal experimental design, Buletinul Institutului Politehnic din Iasi, LVII (LXI), Fasc. 3., 2011, p.149-155.

[41] United States Pharmacopoeia 32, National Formulary 27, New York, 2009, p.1013 (accessed 4 May 2012)

[42] Vijai K., Divya T. Dissolution in Remington The Science and Practice of Pharmacy, 21st ed., Lippincott Williams & Wilkins, Maryland, 2006, p.687.

[43] Yixin C., Tianjie J., McCall, T.W., Baichwal R.A., Meyer C.M. Comparison of Four Artificial Neural Network Software Programs Used to Predict the In Vitro Dissolution of Controlled-Release Tablets, Pharmaceutical Development and Technology, 2002;7(3), 373-379.

[44] Beyssac E., Lavigne J. Dissolution study of active pharmaceutical ingredients using the flow through apparatus USP 4. Dissolution Technol., 2005;12, 23-25.

[45] Ocana J., Frutos G, Sanchez O. Using the similarity factors in practice: A critical revision and suggestions for its standard error estimation. Chemometrics and Intelligent Laboratory Systems, 99 (1), 2009; 49-56.

[46] Maggio R.M., Castellano P.M., Kaufman T.S. A new principal component analysis-based approach for testing "similarity" of drug dissolution profiles. European Journal of Pharmaceutical Sciences, 34(1), 2008: 66-77.

[47] Costa P., Sousa J.M. Lobo Modeling and comparison of dissolution profiles. European Journal of Pharmaceutical Sciences, 13(2), 2001; 123-133.

[48] Chaubal M. Using chitosan as an excipient for oral drug delivery. Drug Deliv. Tech. 2003;3 (3): article 1.

[49] Mao S., Shuai X., Unger F., Simon M., Bi D., Kissel T. The depolymerization of chitosan: Effects on physicochemical and biological properties. Int J Pharm 2004;281, 45-54.

[50] Giunchedi P., Juliano C., Gavini E., Cossu M., Sorrenti M. Formulation and in vivo evaluation of chlorhexidine buccal tablets prepared using drug-loaded chitosan microspheres. Eur. J. Pharm. 2002;53, 233-239.

[51] Bernkop-Schnurch A. Chitosan and its derivates: Potential excipients for peroral peptide delivery systems. Int. J. Pharm. 2000;194, 1-13.

[52] Bernkop-Schnurch A., Krajicek M.E. Mucoadhesive polymers as platforms for peroral peptide delivey and absorption: Syntesis and evaluation of different chitosan-EDTA conjugates. J. Control. Rel. 1998;50, 215-223.

[53] Dodane V., Khan M.A., Merwin J.R, Effect of chitosan on epithelial permeability and structure. Int. J. Pharm. 1999;182, 21-32.

[54] Kotze A.F., Lueßen H.L., De Boer A.G., Verhoef J.C., Junginger H.E. Chitosan for enhanced intestinal permeability: Prospects for derivates soluble in neutral and basic environments. Eur. J. Pharm. 1998;7, 145-151.

[55] Thanou M.M., Kotze A.F., Scharringhausen T,. Lussen H.L., De Boer A.G., Verhoef J.C., Junginger H.E., Effect of degree of quaterization of N-trimethyl chitosan chlor-

ide for enhanced transport of hydrophilic compounds across intestinal Caco-2 cell monolayers.J Controlled Rel 2000; 64, 15-25.

[56] Kotzé A.F., Thanou M.M., Lueben H.L., De Boer A.G., Verhoef J.C., Junginger H.E. Enhancement of paracellular drug transport with highly quaternized N-trimethylchitosan chloride in neutral environments: In vitro evaluation in intestinal epithelial cells (Caco-2). J Pharm Sci 1999; 88, 253-257.

[57] Hamman J.H., Schultz C.M., Kotze A.F. N-trimethyl chitosan chloride: optimum degree of quaternization for drug absorption enhancement across epithelial cells. Drug Dev Ind Pharm 2003; 29, 161-172.

[58] Mao H., Roy K., Troung-Le V.L., Janes K.A., Lin K.Y., Wang Y., August J.T., Leong K.W. Chitosan-DNA nanoparticles as gene carriers: synthesis, characterization and transfection efficiency. J Controlled Rel 2001; 70, 399-421.

[59] Costa P., Lobo J.M.S. Modeling and comparison of dissolution profiles. Eur. J. Pharm. Sci.,13, 2001, p.123.

[60] Avachat A., Kotwal V. Design and evaluation of matrix-based controlled release tablets of diclofenac sodium and chondroitin sulphate, AAPS PharmSciTech, 8, nr.4, 2007, article 88.

[61] Saeio K., Pongpaibul Y., Viernstein S.O. Factors influencing drug dissolution characteristic from hydrophilic polymer matrix tablet, Sci. Pharm., 75, 2007, p.147.

[62] Maderuelo C, Zarzuelo A, Lanao JM. Critical factors in the release of drugs from sustained release hydrophilic matrices. J Control Release. 2011;154, 2-19.

[63] Singh SK, Pandit JK, Mishra DN. Formulation and *in vitro* evaluation of carbopol 934P matrix tablets: Influence of drug solubility and co-excipients on release rate of the drug. J Pharm Res. 2007;6, 20-4.

[64] Singh SK, Pandit JK, Mishra DN. Influence of drug solubility, drug polymer ratio, nature of co-excipients and thermal treatment on drug release from carbopol 974P matrix tablet. Acta Pharma Sciencia. 2006;48, 167-78.

[65] Singh SK, Vijay Kumar SG, Pandit JK, Mishra DN. HPMC based matrix tablet of nimodipine: Effect of viscosity of polymer, type of diluents and sintering on *in vitro* release. J Sci Pharm. 2006;7, 101-9.

[66] Fosamax® (alendronate sodium) package insert, Merck&Co.Inc., 2008, accessed via the internet at http://www.merck.com/product/Fosamax (accessed 3 February 2014).

[67] Fulya K., Nevin C. Bisphosphonates and alendronate, J. Phar,. Sci., 2006;31, 31-42.

[68] Orcel P., Beaudreuil J., Bisphosphonates in bone diseases other than osteoporosis. Joint Bone Spine, 2002;69, 19-27.

[69] Tsun E.C., Heck A.M. Intermittent dosing of alendronate, Ann Pharmacother, 2001;35, 1471-1475.

[70] Porras A.G., Holland S.D., Gertz B.J. Pharmacokinetics of alendronate, Clin Pharmacokinet, 1999;36(5), 315-328.

[71] Stepensky D., Golomb G., Hoffman A. Pharmacokinetic and pharmacodynamic evaluation of intermittent versus continuous alendronate administration in rats, J Pharm Sci. 2002;91(2), 508-516.

[72] Akcay T., Turan S., Guran T., Bereket A. Alendronate Treatment in Children with Osteogenesis Imperfecta, Indian Pediatrics 2008; 45, 105-109.

[73] Hirabayashi H., Fujisaki J., Bone – Specific Drug Delivery Systems Approaches via Chemical Modification of Bine Seeking Agents, Clin Pharmacokinet 2003; 42 (15), 1319-1330.